Public Interest, Private Decisions

KT-433-699

HEALTH-RELATED RESEARCH IN THE UK

ANTHONY HARRISON
BILL NEW

The King's Fund is an independent charitable foundation working for better health, especially in London. We carry out research, policy analysis and development activities, working on our own, in partnerships, and through grants. We are a major resource to people working in health, offering leadership and education courses; seminars and workshops; publications; information and library services; a specialist bookshop; and conference and meeting facilities.

Published by
King's Fund
11–13 Cavendish Square
London W1G 0AN
www.kingsfund.org.uk

© King's Fund 2002

Charity registration number: 207401

First published 2002

ISBN 1 85717 467 4

A CIP catalogue record for this book is available from the British Library

Available from:

King's Fund Bookshop
11–13 Cavendish Square
London W1G 0AN
Tel: 020 7307 2591
Fax: 020 7307 2801
www.kingsfundbookshop.org.uk

Edited by Nicola Bennett-Jones
Cover design by Minuche Mazumdar Farrar
Typeset by Grasshopper Design Company
Printed and bound in Great Britain

Outline

Contents

List of figures and tables

Figures

Tables

Abbreviations

ABPI	Association of the British Pharmaceutical Industry
AMRC	Association of Medical Research Charities
CAM	Complementary and Alternative Medicines
CHD	Coronary Heart Disease
CRDC	Central Research and Development Committee
DH	Department of Health (in some quotations)
DHSS	Department of Health and Social Security
DoH	Department of Health (in some quotations)
DRD	Director of Research and Development
DTI	Department of Trade and Industry
ESRC	Economic and Social Research Council
HEA	Health Education Authority
HEFCE	Higher Education Funding Council for England
HTA	Health Technology Assessment
MRC	Medical Research Council
NCCHTA	National Co-ordinating Centre for HTA
NCRI	National Cancer Research Institute
NEAT	New and Emerging Technologies
NHSE	National Health Service Executive
NHSTA	National Health Service Training Authority
NICE	National Institute for Clinical Excellence
OECD	Organisation for Economic Co-operation and Development
OST	Office of Science and Technology
PFI	Private Finance Initiative
R&D	Research and Development
RAE	Research Assessment Exercise (in universities)
RCT	Randomised Control Trial
RDRD	Regional Director of Research and Development
SCPR	Social and Community Planning Research (SCPR)
SDO	Service Delivery and Organisation (SDO)
SET	Science, Engineering and Technology
SGUMDER	Standing Group on University Medical and Dental Education and Research
SIFT	Service Increment for Teaching
SIFTR	Service Increment for Teaching and Research
UCG	University Grants Committee

About the authors

Anthony Harrison is a visiting fellow at the King's Fund; Bill New is an independent researcher. They are the authors of numerous studies in health care policy, including a joint examination of government policy on waiting lists: *Access to elective care: what should really be done about waiting lists*, published by the King's Fund.

Acknowledgements

The authors are grateful for comments on early drafts from John Appleby and Jonathan Grant, for the substantial contribution made to the clarity of the text by its editor, Nicola Bennett-Jones, and for the publishing support from the Corporate Affairs team at the King's Fund.

Preface

The NHS is, or should be, a knowledge-based service: doctors and other professionals undergo extensive training to ensure they are fit to practise and large sums are devoted, in this country and elsewhere in the developed world, to the search for new forms of treatment.

But over a decade ago, a report from the House of Lords Science and Technology Committee concluded that the NHS itself was *not* getting the knowledge it needed. The vast majority of the research being carried out in NHS hospitals, universities and Government-owned laboratories, not to mention the private sector, did not contribute to solving the problems faced by those working in the NHS on a day-to-day basis, such as how best to manage waiting lists or to provide emergency care. Nor did it bear on the longer-term issues which any health service has to resolve:

- What should the balance be between hospital and community services?
- How large should hospitals be and what range of functions should they carry out?
- What should the contribution of public health measures be relative to health care itself?

The then Government responded vigorously to these criticisms. A Directorate of Research and Development was established within the Department of Health, charged with the task of creating a better match between the needs of the service and the research being carried out within the NHS itself and the broader research community.

Over the last decade, a series of policies have been introduced, covering finance and the selection of projects, aimed at discharging this task. New programmes have been established to focus on previously neglected areas.

But the supply side of the health research economy has proved problematic outside the medical field. Here there is a chicken-and-egg problem: expansion of research in these areas has been hindered by the lack of trained professionals and appropriate institutions. But universities seeking to develop these can make their case, in the current environment, only if they have a good track record in the first place. Again a number of policies have been brought in to try to remove this obstacle.

While it is clearly important that research funded by the Department of Health and the NHS, now costing about £500 million a year, should be properly targeted, it represents only a fraction of total research expenditure bearing on health. Other parts of the public sector such as the research councils and the universities spend more in total. Not-for-profit organisations such as Cancer UK account for a further £500 million. But all these are outweighed by spending within the private sector, mainly by pharmaceutical and biotechnology companies. Their spending is now running at some £3 billion a year and is rapidly rising. Furthermore, very much larger sums are being spent worldwide in the search for new drugs and other forms of treatment.

This health research economy is driven by a variety of forces. Within the private sector, profit is the major driver and it is underpinned by the patent system. But choice of research programmes across all sectors is strongly influenced by prevailing scientific opinion and the professional interests of those engaged in research. This leads to the question: does this mix of incentives and constraints ensure that the research being funded offers the greatest possible chance of improving health and, in particular, meeting the needs of the NHS as a deliverer of care? And if it does not, what means are available to bring public health and private interests into line?

The evidence suggests that the current balance of research reflects a number of biases within the health research economy and hence that certain kinds of research attract little, if any, funding. Research in some areas is unlikely to be profitable because the results cannot be patented; others areas are of little scientific interest.

The large role played by the not-for-profit sector goes some way towards redressing the resulting imbalances but, large though it is by international standards, this sector cannot be relied upon to ensure that the health research economy best serves the NHS and its patients.

The current mechanisms for orchestrating the various elements of the health research economy into an effective whole are limited in scope. While various measures have been taken to bring into line the work of the

Medical Research Council (MRC), the universities and the private sector, the available mechanisms are only partially effective, depending as they do largely on co-ordination and communication rather than direction.

Since the challenge was posed by the House of Lords report, the world itself has changed. At that time, only a little over a decade ago, the professional was still assumed to know best. But increasingly that assumption is being rejected. Recent controversies over BSE, food safety in general and MMR have revealed that the public does not necessarily accept what the professional and scientific community tells it. Official advice may therefore be rejected, while many turn to remedies outside the realm of conventional medicine. This poses a new challenge: how can the research community as a whole retain the trust of those it is intended to serve.

A decade or so after the R&D initiative was established, it is time to take stock of how successful it has been. This book therefore assesses how much progress has been made towards achieving a better match between the needs of the NHS and the work being supported by the Department of Health within and outside the NHS.

It then goes on to consider how the role of such publicly financed research should be defined, given the parts played by the universities, the for-profit sector and the not-for-profit sector.

Finally it assesses the significance of the change in public attitudes towards science in general and health research in particular.

This study represents a development of Chapter 10 of *The NHS: Facing the future* (Harrison and Dixon, 2000) written by one of the present authors (Anthony Harrison) and Jennifer Dixon. That chapter posed the question: Does the NHS have available to it the knowledge base it requires? The present study offers a more detailed consideration of the same question.

Anthony Harrison
Bill New

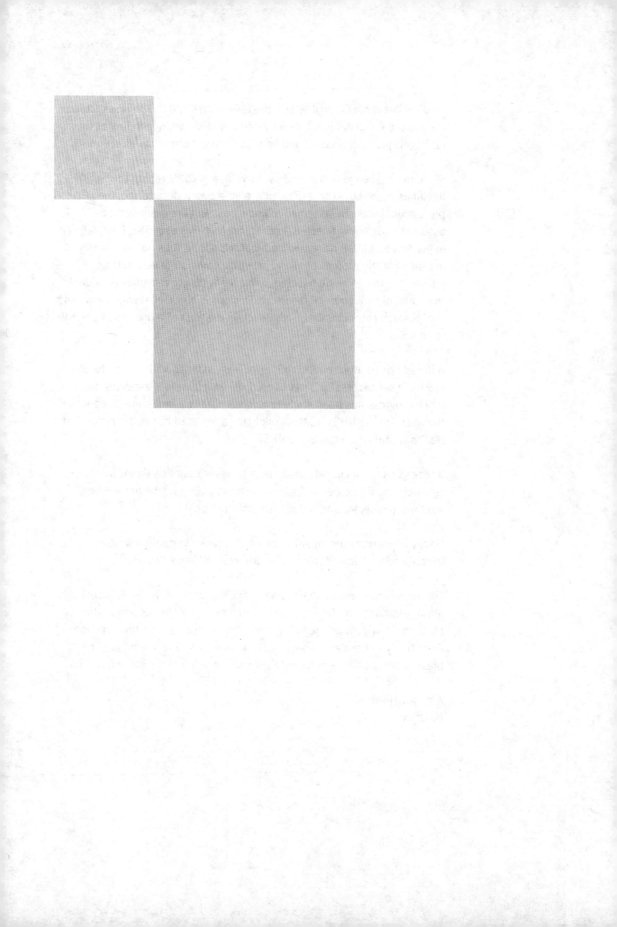

Introduction

The central question posed in this study is 'Do we get the best "bundle" of knowledge out of the resources devoted to health-related R&D?'. This introductory chapter points to issues to be considered in answering that question: criticisms of health-related research, the role of the public sector and the relationship between the health research economy and the general public.

Introduction

For a century or more it has been accepted that the delivery of health care should be based on 'knowledge'. After the passing of the 1858 Medical Act, the practice of medicine was limited to those with formal qualifications. By the early 20th century, following 'the bacteriological revolution ... medicine wedded itself not only to science but became the great incorporator of knowledge' (Illich *et al.*, 1977, p.48). As a result, modern medical knowledge, according to Wright and Treacher, has been characterised by two features:

> it was built upon the findings of modern science; and it was effective. Its scientific foundation was important because medicine drew from it the same privileged epistemological status that was usually accorded to science: if science was the accurate reading of Nature's book with eyes undistorted by social interest or cultural prejudice, medicine was the benevolent application of some of what was found there. The history of medicine, in consequence, was frequently expressed in triumphalist terms: as a process of refining; of separating the pure, neutral, scientific essence from everything that had contaminated it.

> Wright and Treacher, 1982, p.4

Consequently:

> what ultimately distinguished medicine was that it possessed a core of veracious knowledge about the natural world which was distinct from anything social.

> Wright and Treacher 1982, p.5

For the last century or so, the main route to 'veracious knowledge' has been systematically organised scientific and clinical research carried out within hospitals or public and private research establishments devoted to medicine or broader-based science.

Worldwide, perhaps as much as $80 billion is devoted to medical research each year, of which over $7 billion is spent in the UK (Global Forum for Health Research, 2002). The results of this research have led to rapid technical change – new drugs, new treatments and new equipment – which has vastly expanded the range of what the NHS can do and the number of people who can benefit from clinical care (Bunker, 2001). The prospect is that technical change will continue and, if anything, be more rapid (Sykes, 2000).

Criticisms of health-related research

Although health-related research continues to attract an increasing share of national economic and scientific resources, and despite the prospect of improvements to health and well being that it holds out, it has increasingly been criticised on a number of fronts:

- Despite the scale of expenditure, some health care needs attract very little attention and particular diseases are neglected. The overwhelming emphasis in current research is on drugs and other procedures, rather than on the often complex processes involved in the actual delivery of and the management of health care systems as a whole.
- Too little attention is paid to the causes and prevention of ill health so that health systems are condemned to be 'sickness' systems, dealing with the consequences of disease.
- Most research ignores the range of approaches lumped together as complementary and alternative medicine, which are not deemed to be 'scientific'. Equally, alternative approaches within the ambit of conventional medical science may be ignored by grant givers, and peer reviewers view them as 'unsound'.
- The potential for the user also to be a provider of care and the contribution of carers and lay advisers to their own care or that of others are underestimated.
- The drive for greater and greater understanding of basic physiological processes throws up more and more difficult ethical dilemmas, such as those arising from the use of stem cells from embryos, of a kind which society finds difficult to grapple with.
- The trend towards medicalisation of an ever-wider range of problems is ultimately self-defeating, making people more and more dependent on increasingly expensive services. Health care, in other words, is itself a kind of addictive drug, at least for some.

We have set out these criticisms roughly along the spectrum: starting with the tactical and ending with the fundamental (Illich, 1975). Different types of question can be raised at different points along this spectrum.

1 **SPECTRUM OF CRITICISMS OF HEALTH RESEARCH**		
TACTICAL	INTERMEDIATE	FUNDAMENTAL
Does the current balance of effort in research accurately reflect the needs of those seeking care from a health service organised more or less as it is now?	Do the research methods which currently attract most funding represent the only or best way of producing knowledge?	Can we put faith in the medical enterprise at all?

This study will not consider the criticisms at the fundamental end of the spectrum (the last two bullet points above), but it will address the tactical and intermediate criticisms. In other words, it accepts that the provision of health care should based on the results of formally organised research. This is not to say that health care can or should be based exclusively on such research: judgements made by clinicians and managers are inevitably based on experience, intuition and their interactions with those they treat or whose work they direct (Higgs and Titchen, 2001). In many cases they are confronted with uncertainty and risk which research cannot dispel.

The same is true of individuals making decisions about their own health and care, of politicians considering whether to promote change in the organisation of care and the population at large faced with the prospect of such change. In fields such as this, research cannot promise certainty that the right decisions will be taken. Furthermore, as decisions affecting the health care system involve choosing between benefits accruing to different groups of people, they necessarily involve value rather than scientific judgements. Even here, however, evidence, argument and information may be brought to bear. Such decisions also fall within the compass of this study.

The central question

Despite the central role played by health-related R&D in the development of the NHS – and other health care systems – the present pattern of spending in the UK and elsewhere is not the result of the coherent and consistent pursuit of knowledge relevant to the 'health of the nation' or 'the needs of the NHS'. Rather, different interest groups, particularly the medical profession, parts of the scientific world and the private sector, have been able to command resources to realise, at least in part, their own view of what constitutes the best approach to producing relevant knowledge.

Others within the medical field, including professions such as nursing, whose views are treated as unorthodox and those who promote non-medical solutions to what are currently perceived as medical problems have found it harder to influence the production of knowledge. So, too, have the ultimate beneficiaries, the users of health services.

The central question with which this study is concerned therefore is:

> Do we get the best 'bundle' of knowledge out of the resources currently devoted to health-related R&D?

The corollary of this question is another one: Are there biases or constraints in the way the health research is conducted, which lead to important areas being systematically neglected and less important areas being intensively researched?

Given the importance of technical progress to the development of the NHS and health care systems across the world, it might be expected that these questions would have been a major preoccupation of policy makers. But for most of the history of the NHS questions about the scale and balance of R&D spending within and for the NHS have been largely ignored in public debate or even informed analysis – R&D merited just one thin paragraph in the Labour Government's first white paper. Technical progress has been regarded as a 'given', welcome because of the new treatments it provides, but less welcome because of its implications for the overall budget (Wanless, 2001).

This lack of questioning is in part explained by the role played by the private sector. In the context of its economic and industrial policies, the

Government has a strong interest in the success of the private sector as a producer of wealth. In the context of health policy, its interest lies in the contribution of privately financed research to new and better forms of treatment. As a result, Government policy is pulled in two directions. The tension is clear in these two extracts from the Department of Health policy paper, *Research and Development for a First Class Service*:

> *2.1 The Government works to improve the wealth, health and well being of the nation. It is committed to modernising the NHS and to improving the quality of the care it provides. Research is vital to these endeavours. Basic and strategic research underpins the development of new ways of promoting and protecting health and curing and caring for the sick. Applied research underpins improvements in the organisation, responsiveness, effectiveness and efficiency of services.*
>
> *2.2 The Government also promotes science, technology and technology transfer to improve the competitiveness of industry and the quality of public services. It wishes to maintain and improve the UK's international standing in science in general and biomedical science in particular. To this end, it seeks to promote the partnership within and between government, the NHS, the universities, industry and the voluntary sector that will allow health related research to prosper and ensure that the nation continues to reap the benefits to health and wealth that such work can bring.*
>
> Department of Health, 2000b, p.9

The sentiments expressed in these two paragraphs are unremarkable and in themselves would provoke little dissent. However, they contain the seeds of conflict. The competitiveness of UK industry and its international standing in bioscience is primarily a matter of wealth rather than health creation; the needs of public services, primarily the NHS, are concerned with health rather than wealth. The two broad policy objectives overlap, but do not completely coincide. Measures to promote UK competitiveness may yield no health benefits, and measures to promote UK health may yield no industrial benefits.

The role of the public sector

In this study we are concerned solely with the production of health benefits and therefore do not consider how well the current pattern of R&D spending serves the interests of the national economy. Nor do we address the question of whether the vast sums spent by the pharmaceutical industry in drug development are 'well spent' from the viewpoint of health service users. Instead we focus on what the role of the public sector should be, given the nature of the private sector.

But the role of the private sector is nevertheless central to what follows. As the major spender on health-related R&D, what it does is of critical importance to the promotion of health, particularly in those areas such as the development of new drugs and medical devices where its role is dominant. But just as important is the question of what it does *not* do. If there are areas of research which the private sector will not fund and if those areas might produce substantial health benefits, then there is a strong *prima facie* case for the public sector to finance research into them or to encourage, through financial or other incentives, the private sector to do so.

Although that may seem obvious enough, the starting point for this study is the presumption that the public sector does not fulfil this role. This presumption stems from a report from the House of Lords Science and Technology Committee published in 1988 (House of Lords, 1988). The report concluded that the pattern of spending on health-related research by the public sector ignored many important research areas, in particular the needs of the NHS as a deliverer of care. While the Committee did not expect to find that private sector funding research was designed to improve the NHS as a deliverer of care, it did expect to find that publicly funded research, or a substantial part of it, had that focus. It found, however, that it did not.

Since the publication of the House of Lords report, health research coming under the direction of the Department of Health has received sustained attention from policy makers. Like the NHS itself it has been subject to a process of continuous revolution largely designed to meet the criticisms made in the 1988 report. This process of reform is the main focus of this study.

The process began with the publication of *Research for Health* (Department of Health, 1991a), the first policy response to the House of

Lords' criticisms. Since then, and right up to the present, there has been a stream of official papers setting out further reforms of the management of centrally funded research and of the arrangements for bringing together the various contributors to health research.

Questioning the authority of professionals

While the reform process has been under way, however, other developments have worked to undermine the central features of medical authority identified by Wright and Treacher above. Of these, the most important is the changing role of the ultimate customer of the research, the user of health care services.

Health research is by its nature almost entirely a professional affair. Its authority rests on the nature of the discoveries and inventions it has produced using techniques of investigation, concepts and theories far beyond the capacity of ordinary citizens and indeed of most frontline professionals. The last ten years have seen rapid growth in mechanisms designed to assess the results of this work, to bring out their relevance to clinical practice and to encourage as appropriate their application in the day-to-day delivery of care.[1]

These developments have revealed that the implicit claims to authority underlying medical practice are frequently not justified. Treatments are rejected, clinical guidelines revised and procedures once deemed safe are banned because of the risks they pose to patients. This process can be seen as part and parcel of taking evidence seriously, with the resulting recommendations commanding more authority by virtue of the methods used for deriving them.

But there may be differences in professional opinion. Where experts disagree and their differences are fully aired in public, as they were during the BSE crisis for example, the basis of 'authority' is undermined. Given the complexity of the science involved, attempts to demonstrate safety or otherwise inevitably have to be left to those with relevant expertise. In this particular case, it became apparent that, although the experts knew more than anyone else, they did not know enough to be sure that 'eating beef was safe' or precisely what degree of risks it posed.

---

1. These include the Cochrane collaborations which are now worldwide, new journals and, in the UK, the National Institute for Clinical Excellence.

Some years later, the same issue arose over the safety or otherwise of the triple MMR vaccine: the official line was challenged by a small number of researchers, leaving parents uncertain as to which advice to follow. Although most parents appear to have followed the official line, many did not. In this case the authority of the State as a proponent of the triple vaccine rests on the authority of science: threats to the latter are inevitably threats to the former as well.

In these cases, politicians and the public had to deal with events as they arose. But a great deal of research is planned and executed over a long time period. What is the public's role here? It is now becoming conventional, when it comes to treatment, to use the language of professional–patient partnership (Kennedy, 2001), meaning that decisions on treatment and care should be made jointly by professionals and patients in dialogue together. Within the field of R&D, the user voice is only just beginning to be heard. So far, that voice is faint, and the notion of partnership has yet fully to take hold. But if the NHS is to be built round its users, so should the research which supports it and, as we shall see, the priorities of users are not identical to those of professionals.

We have posed the question: Do we get the best 'bundle' of knowledge out of the resources devoted to health-related R&D? In the last analysis this is a question about values and hence a matter for citizens rather than experts. Although the process of research is inevitably largely a professional matter, deciding what areas to investigate is not: whether such decisions are made by professionals, politicians or lay people, they entail value judgements. Our study concludes, therefore, with a consideration of possible changes in the way health-related research is run, which would reflect change in the context in which such research is carried out.

Outline of this study

The focus of this study is what we term the 'health research economy'. We use this term to refer to those parts of the private and public sectors which generate knowledge and information bearing on the wide range of decisions that the provision of a national health service entails. Clearly, the vast majority of the decisions made in the course of delivering NHS services are clinical in nature. But many are concerned with the organisation of services, their location and the buildings they require, the provision of supporting services and technologies and the way in which they are financed and held accountable. In addition a vast range of decisions fall outside the NHS itself: health and safety at work, the control of carcinogenic materials, the provision of basic services such as clean water and housing, the provision of food and many others.

It follows that the health research economy is both very extensive and very diverse. While the main features can be readily described, its precise scope is impossible to set out, because so many organisations, both public and private, make a contribution to it. Furthermore in some fields of knowledge, research may primarily be aimed at other targets, but may have a spin-off for the health economy.

In Chapter 1, therefore, we focus only on the main players in the health research economy as it stands now in the UK – the pharmaceutical industry, the not-for-profit or charitable sector (which is particularly important in health research) and the various contributors from the public sector.

We then consider how the health research economy works. It is not a market in the ordinary sense: instead it consists of a range of public and private organisations with different economic characteristics and faced with different constraints and incentives. In Chapter 2 we focus on two main issues: first, what incentives and biases these organisations (and those working in them) are subject to, and second, how the role of the different elements should be determined. This analysis identifies a range of potential strengths and weaknesses for each of the main participants. In particular it identifies areas where the role of the public sector is likely to be critical in determining how well the health research economy as a whole works.

We go on to describe the attempts that have been made, largely in the last ten years, to redesign that part of the health research economy which lies within the NHS and the control of the Department of Health. Although this represents only a small part of the total health research economy, it is the part over which public policy has, potentially at least, the greatest degree of control. Chapters 3 to 6 consider the attempts which have been made to:

- improve the system for allocating research funds controlled by the Department of Health and the NHS
- make publicly funded research more relevant to the NHS (and to a lesser extent to Government policy making)

- ensure that the supply of research matches the needs for it
- improve the links between the various players in the system and to define their separate roles.

In Chapter 7 we take two conditions – cancer and Parkinson's disease – to assess how the biases, gaps and other failures have affected research in these two areas.

We go on to consider the broader social context surrounding the production of knowledge. As we noted above, the context in which knowledge is produced is changing. Until recently the implicit assumption has been that the knowledge produced is definitive and, where it is not, disputes should be settled within the professional arena. Now users are questioning the basis on which expert judgements are made. In Chapter 8 we consider the implications of this for the relationship between the general public and the producers of knowledge and their immediate market, the health care professionals.

The final chapter assesses the progress that has been made in managing the health research economy in recent years and then goes on to consider what should be done to devise a better system.

Chapter 1

The health research economy: the players and their roles

There are many players in the UK's health research economy, most of them both paying for research and providing it, and all linked to the others in a complex web of relationships. Taking the payer and provider sides in turn, this chapter outlines the roles of the main players – the private sector, charities and the various contributors from the public sector.

1 The health research economy: the players and their roles

This chapter sets out the main features of the health research economy. Following what has become the conventional approach, we divide players into payers and providers. The term 'payers' is carefully chosen, for in general the publicly financed part of the health research economy is simply financed from the exchequer, albeit via indirect routes. Only parts of it are subject to a purchasing or commissioning process of the kind which has been introduced to health care services involving actual or implicit contracts for closely specified pieces of work.

Many of the participants in the health research economy are both payers and providers, which mean that they are more interdependent than the simple division between purchasing and providing suggests. Furthermore, as we shall see, there are strong links between some of the players on the provider side. But for the moment we leave these complexities to one side and consider the two roles separately.

Who pays?

The health research economy has six main components: two private and four public. The private payers comprise the for-profit sector and the not-for-profit, or charitable, sector. The main public payers are the Department of Health, the NHS, the MRC (and to a much smaller extent the other research councils) and the university sector (for which the main funder is the Higher Education Funding Council for England – HEFCE – and its counterparts in the other parts of the UK). Their contributions are set out overleaf.

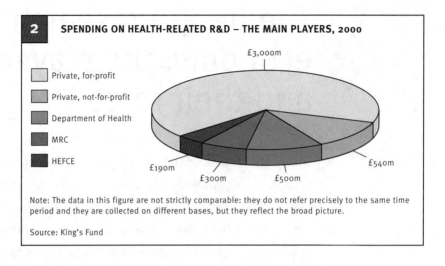

2   **SPENDING ON HEALTH-RELATED R&D – THE MAIN PLAYERS, 2000**

- Private, for-profit
- Private, not-for-profit
- Department of Health
- MRC
- HEFCE

£3,000m

£190m

£300m

£500m

£540m

Note: The data in this figure are not strictly comparable: they do not refer precisely to the same time period and they are collected on different bases, but they reflect the broad picture.

Source: King's Fund

When the House of Lords surveyed the health research economy in 1988, it found that funding was dominated by the private, for-profit, sector. As Figure 2 shows, that remains true now.[2]

The Department of Health and the NHS

The Department of Health funds research for its own use and provides the finance for the NHS's own research programmes. The former comprise the Policy Research, the Health Technology Assessment (HTA), Service Delivery and Organisation (SDO) and the New and Emerging Technologies (NEAT) programmes[3] and the research carried out within the Public Health Laboratory Service and other agencies for which it is accountable. Some

---

2. In 1988 there was very little information available about the scale of spending within the NHS itself, a situation which remained true when the House of Lords prepared a further report in 1995 (House of Lords, 1995). Since then developments, to be described in Chapter 3, have led to a much closer identification of what the NHS spends. Furthermore, developments in science policy during the 1990s have led to a sustained interest in the level of R&D spending across the economy as a whole. As a result, the Office of Science and Technology now publishes annual estimates of R&D spending by main industrial sectors; we rely heavily on these in what follows.

3. HTA attempts to answer questions such as 'Does this treatment work, at what cost and how does it compare with others?'. It is also developing more capacity to undertake 'fast-track' assessments for, e.g. NICE. SDO aims to provide knowledge about how the organisation and delivery of services can be improved to increase the quality of patient care, ensure better strategic outcomes and contribute to improved health. NEAT exists to promote and support, through applied research, the use of new or emerging technologies to develop health care products, the main purpose being to overcome a development barrier and also a perceived 'funding gap'.

of the funding available to these programmes and agencies is allocated in turn to universities and others in the form of project or programme grants, including a number of dedicated units devoted to research in particular topics or disciplines.

NHS funding provides financial support for NHS providers to cover 'excess' or 'service support' costs (not treatment or research costs) of research conducted in NHS providers and of relevance to the NHS, but funded from a variety of sources including research councils and charities. It also finances R&D carried out within the NHS itself by NHS staff, often in combination with other duties such as the day-to-day provision of care. Such research is concentrated in large teaching hospitals, but small amounts of funding are allocated widely across other parts of the NHS.

As Figure 3 (which reflects the situation in the mid-1990s) shows, the bulk of the budget goes to the support of research funded by other parts of the health research economy – particularly the private, not-for-profit sector, which accounts for over a quarter of it. Centrally run programmes account for only 6 per cent, and regionally run programmes for 12 per cent. Just under a fifth goes on research led by the NHS itself.

Office of Science and Technology and the Medical Research Council

The principal and oldest public institution in the field of medical research is the Medical Research Council. It was originally set up as the Medical Research Committee in 1913, and was incorporated under its present title by Royal Charter in 1920. Its purpose, as set out in its Royal Charter, is:

- to encourage and support high-quality research with the aim of maintaining and improving human health
- to train skilled people, and to advance and disseminate knowledge and technology with the aim of meeting national needs in terms of health, quality of life and economic competitiveness
- to promote public engagement with medical research.

Like all research councils, the MRC is funded from a grant-in-aid through the Office of Science and Technology, which itself forms part of the Department of Trade and Industry. The MRC's budget is currently approximately £300 million. Although the MRC has a large in-house

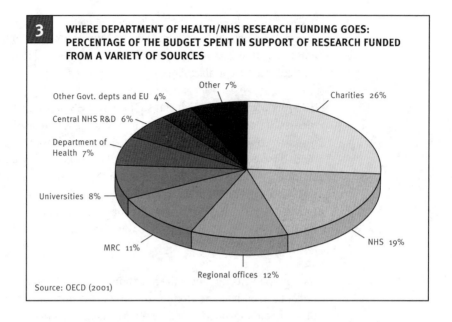

3 WHERE DEPARTMENT OF HEALTH/NHS RESEARCH FUNDING GOES: PERCENTAGE OF THE BUDGET SPENT IN SUPPORT OF RESEARCH FUNDED FROM A VARIETY OF SOURCES

Other 7%
Other Govt. depts and EU 4%
Central NHS R&D 6%
Department of Health 7%
Universities 8%
MRC 11%
Regional offices 12%
NHS 19%
Charities 26%

Source: OECD (2001)

research capacity, it also funds research by means of a range of external grants. These include administrative support for the Institute of Cancer Research and Strangeways Research Laboratory, a number of programme grants to support the long-term work of university research departments and project grants which are designed to provide support for a specific piece of work. Finally it supports the training of researchers through fellowships and studentships. The table below sets out its main areas of work and the proportion of its budget attached to each.

Other research councils also contribute to the health research economy. The range of the councils' work is so wide that we have not attempted to

TABLE 1: MRC RESEARCH AND TRAINING SPEND BY SCIENTIFIC FIELD

SCIENTIFIC FIELD	% OF BUDGET
Neuroscience and mental health	18
Immunology and infection	18
Medical physiology and disease processes	18
Cell biology, development and growth	17
Genetics, molecular structure and dynamics	16
People and population studies: health services and the health of the public	13

estimate their contribution to the health research economy. However, it includes the fundamental work carried out by the Biotechnology and Biological Sciences Research Council on genome research and biomolecular science and most recently a new initiative on ageing involving contributions from several councils (see Chapter 4).

As we shall see in Chapter 6, the Department of Health has negotiated concordats with each council, under which information is exchanged. In principle, at least, this encourages the councils to respond to the needs of the NHS by modifying or redirecting the funds at their disposal. However, neither the MRC nor the other research councils are accountable to the Department of Health for their contribution to health research.

The Higher Education Funding Council for England

The HEFCE funds research in the university sector through a block grant which reflects its assessment of the performance of individual institutions in research terms, but which is not formally tied to specific subjects. SET statistics separate out expenditure on five broad subject areas for HEFCE-funded R&D and SET expenditure, as shown in Figure 4.[4]

Clearly medical research funded by the HEFCE counts as part of the health research economy. It is difficult, however, to establish how much more of the total research might be considered relevant to health care R&D. Some research in social science and the humanities as well as engineering and

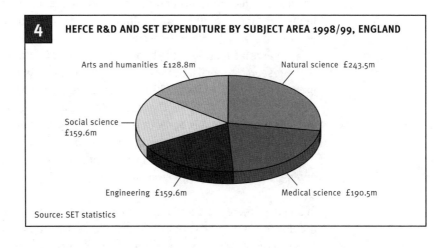

4 **HEFCE R&D AND SET EXPENDITURE BY SUBJECT AREA 1998/99, ENGLAND**

Arts and humanities £128.8m

Natural science £243.5m

Social science — £159.6m

Engineering £159.6m

Medical science £190.5m

Source: SET statistics

4. SET (Science, Engineering and Technology) expenditure is defined as research and experimental development, technology transfer and postgraduate education and training.

natural sciences will contribute to health care, e.g. by the invention of a medical device or providing the basis for an understanding of some of the physical processes in the environment bearing on health. No allowance for possible contributions from these areas has been included in Figure 2.

Other Government departments

A number of other Government departments provide small amounts of support, and in particular fields they may be the main Government funders. There are agencies outside the health care sector such as the Food Standards Agency. There are also Government departments which contribute to the public health agenda and which have research programmes of their own.

For example, the Department of the Environment, Transport and the Regions supports (along with the Department of Health) research into the health effects of air pollution. The Department of Trade and Industry supports work on medical technology through, for example, the Medlink programme and technology transfer programmes such as TCS (formerly the Teaching Company Scheme). The Office of National Statistics has a significant in-house health research programme. The Scottish Executive, the National Assembly for Wales and the Northern Ireland Executive/Office have programmes of their own.

The role of the Department of Trade and Industry and the Office of Science and Technology is particularly important as it intersects with the interests of the Department of Health in the area of 'support for science' and the use by industry of the results of research. As noted, the Office of Science and Technology is the body through which funds are channelled to the research councils. But, in addition, the Department of Trade and Industry runs programmes of its own and forms the focus for Government support for R&D as a whole. The Medlink programme, part-funded by the Department of Health, is part of a larger LINK programme run by the Office of Science and Technology and designed to boost collaborative work within industry across a number of selected areas, including some which impinge on health, e.g. nutrition and ageing.

In addition, there are contributions from publicly funded bodies such as the House of Commons and Lords committees, the Audit Commission, the National Audit Office and more recently the Commission for Health Improvement and NICE. All produce reports which shed a light on how things work in practice and which, because of the unique powers of access of these bodies, no other organisations could produce.

We have not included an estimate of the scale of these various contributions to the health research economy in Figure 2. Although reliable figures are available for some of the above (e.g. the Food Standards Agency has a budget of about £25 million), for many of the others only rough figures could be estimated. However, it seems unlikely that funding all the above taken together exceeds £100 million, and clearly no one agency spends more than a small fraction of the spending of the main players listed in Figure 2.

The table below breaks down public sector R&D spending by main purpose. It suggests that only a small part of the MRC budget is devoted to the support of service delivery and a still smaller amount to technology support. Spending by the Department of Health is largely attributed to policy support and a small amount to technology support. Most spending by the NHS is attributed to service support. However, as noted already, Figure 3 suggests that a high proportion of this figure is in fact used to support research by other contributors to the health research economy.

TABLE 2: ANALYSIS OF NET GOVERNMENT R&D EXPENDITURE IN £m BY PRIMARY PURPOSE AND DEPARTMENT, 1999/2000

	MRC	DEPARTMENT OF HEALTH	NHS
General support	269.6	0.2	0
Service support	32.5	29.0	409.7
Policy support	0.5	31.8	0.2
Technology support	1.2	1.7	0.0
Total R&D	303.7	62.6	409.9

Source: Derived from SET statistics, available at: www.dti.gov.uk

The private contribution

The for-profit sector

As Figure 2 shows, the health research economy is dominated by the private sector.5 The for-profit sector, particularly the pharmaceutical industry, contributes by far the largest component of UK spending on health-related medical research. The Association of the British Pharmaceutical Industry (ABPI) claims that pharmaceutical companies carry out almost 20 per cent of all industrial R&D in Britain, spending more than 20 per cent of their gross output on R&D – a proportion which has risen by some seven percentage points since the mid-1980s.

In Figure 5, total current spending by the private for-profit sector is broken down into broad categories. Not unexpectedly, only a small fraction is deemed to be pure research: the bulk is categorised as developmental.

Much of this research is concentrated in a small number of large companies – indeed some of these spend as much as the whole of the Department of Health R&D budget. However, much smaller companies in the biotechnology sector are now beginning to make significant contributions to the health research economy, but we have not been able

---

5. This is not true of the USA as the following table shows:

Table 3: Funding for health R&D, according to source of funds, USA 1995

Source of funding	$ million
All funding	35,816
Industry	18,645
Private non-profit organisations	1,325
State and Local Governments	2,423
Federal Government	13,423
National Institutes of Health	10,682
National Institute on Aging	419
National Institute of Allergy and Infectious Diseases	1,096
National Cancer Institute	2,084
National Institute of Child Health and Human Development	543
National Institute of Diabetes and Digestive and Kidney Diseases	697
National Institute of Drug Abuse	434
National Institute of General Medical Sciences	783
National Heart, Lung and Blood Institute	1,229
National Institute of Mental Health	591
National Institute of Neurological Disorders and Stroke	633
Other National Institutes of Health	2,172
Other	2,741

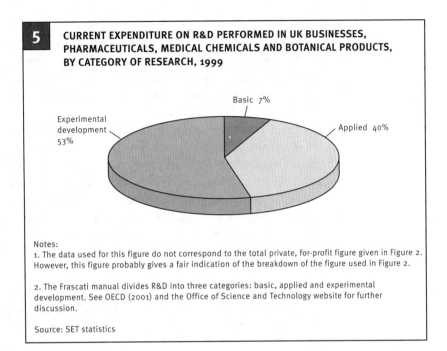

5 CURRENT EXPENDITURE ON R&D PERFORMED IN UK BUSINESSES, PHARMACEUTICALS, MEDICAL CHEMICALS AND BOTANICAL PRODUCTS, BY CATEGORY OF RESEARCH, 1999

Basic 7%

Experimental development 53%

Applied 40%

Notes:
1. The data used for this figure do not correspond to the total private, for-profit figure given in Figure 2. However, this figure probably gives a fair indication of the breakdown of the figure used in Figure 2.

2. The Frascati manual divides R&D into three categories: basic, applied and experimental development. See OECD (2001) and the Office of Science and Technology website for further discussion.

Source: SET statistics

to include a reliable estimate of the scale of spending involved. In addition, the NHS draws on many thousands of companies for medical devices and other equipment required for surgical and other procedures. Information on how much such companies spend on research is not available, but it is safe to assume that it is small relative to the drug companies.

The not-for-profit sector

There are now several hundred charitable bodies supporting health-related research. Virtually all are 'single issue' organisations, which focus on a particular disease or group, such as elderly people. There are also groups which support the production of knowledge in their own locality.

In addition there are bodies such as the King's Fund and the Nuffield Trust which support, or themselves carry out, health-related research. Their contribution lies mainly in the organisation and delivery of care and issues of concern to national policy makers.

Most charities are small. But, in 1998/99, the total amount of money donated from just two of the cancer charities – the Imperial Cancer Research Fund and the Cancer Research Campaign (which have recently merged to form Cancer UK) – was over £100 million.[6] The largest individual contributor is the Wellcome Trust, which accounts for about half of the £540 million shown in Figure 2.[7] The Trust derives its funds from a single large endowment rather than from continuous voluntary giving, and is the only major charity free to fund research in any field.

As noted, most charities focus on particular conditions. Some, like the cancer charities, are concerned with common conditions. However, others support research (and other activities) into much rarer conditions affecting only a small number of people and have only very small budgets at their disposal. The not-for-profit sector is the principal source of funding in a number of areas including cancer, ophthalmology, cystic fibrosis, diabetes, psychiatry and heart disease. In these areas the charities are as much campaigning bodies as research sponsors.

According to the Association of Medical Research Charities (AMRC), the scale of charitable funding for medical research in the UK is 'unparalleled elsewhere in the world'. The broad purposes to which it is devoted are shown in the table opposite.

The AMRC states that it is not possible to make estimates of the share of these resources going to strategic or applied research, but it is safe to say that, although individual charities may focus on one particular part of the spectrum, the sector as a whole supports work ranging from basic science to service development.

TABLE 4: AMRC CHARITIES, EXPENDITURE BY PURPOSE OF THE CHARITY, 1998/99	
PURPOSE OF CHARITY	%
General medical research	45.20
Cancer and leukaemia	30.42
Heart/lung/stroke	11.59
Arthritis and orthopaedics	4.29
Other disease, specific	3.49
Neurology and mental health	2.26
Genetic conditions	1.35
Children and foetal health	0.77
Sight and hearing	0.63

Source: www.amrc.org.uk

---

6. In evidence to the Science and Technology Committee of the House of Commons, Sir John Pattison said that the Government contribution now exceeded that of the not-for-profit sector, but the Committee was not impressed with the figuring: see Chapter 7.

7. In recent years the Wellcome Trust has made major contributions to the development of the UK science base, particularly genomics. Its total budget is therefore much higher than the amount included in Figure 2.

Providers

All the main actors identified, with the exception of the HEFCE, are providers as well as financers of research.

The role of the NHS

The role of the NHS within the provider system is complex and much larger than its modest contribution to the spending total might suggest. It is at one and the same time a provider of research in its own right and a provider of the basic infrastructure for research by others. The 'production' of research is part of a complex system which, within the NHS itself, involves the provision of care and clinical teaching as well as research activity. The patients the NHS treats are a central part of the production process, particularly for the development and testing of new drugs and surgical procedures. Its buildings house research facilities, some if not most funded from outside sources; many of its staff include research among their duties, but that research may be supported by outside funders.

As the House of Lords 1988 report puts it:

> *3.19 The NHS is inextricably involved with medical research. It is responsible for the health of the nation in which research has a vital role. It is the ultimate customer for nearly all medical research, whether funded by the MRC, the charities, the pharmaceutical and medical equipment industries or done in the NHS itself. Practically all clinical research is carried out in NHS hospitals; it involves clinicians on NHS contracts ... NHS nursing and ancillary staff, and NHS patients. Teaching hospitals provide the tertiary referral facilities for many parts of the country because of their academic and clinical strength in various specialties. ... Last, but by no means least, the resources on which clinical medical and dental education are based are the NHS's responsibility.*

The hospital is the locus where these three elements of research, teaching and care intersect. Historically in the UK and elsewhere the teaching and research hospital has been at the centre of the health research economy – indeed its driving force. Even now, only a small number of UK hospitals are significant providers of research: most is carried out within the older-established institutions.

The private for-profit and not-for-profit sectors taken together command much larger budgets than all the public sources combined, and to a large degree they are independent of the public sector, able as they are to decide for themselves how much they spend on what. But the private sector requires access to NHS patients and in some cases NHS researchers and clinicians for scientific work and above all clinical trials. To meet these needs the NHS requires a physical and human infrastructure with the necessary scientific and organisational skills to be in a position to work in effective collaboration with the private sector as well as with publicly funded researchers. As Figure 3 (p.18) shows, this support function represents a significant claim on NHS resources.

The importance of this distinction between the provision of infrastructure for research by others and 'own account' research by the NHS has emerged over the last few years both in general and in relation to particular diseases such as cancer. Until recently, it has not been fully recognised in the way that funding has been allocated to NHS providers, but from 2002 onwards it will be reflected in a distribution formula which distinguishes the support role from the execution of in-house research (see Chapter 3).

The Medical Research Council

The MRC employs research staff at its own major research establishment, the National Institute for Medical Research at Mill Hill, and at 53 research units, most of which are close to or within a university or hospital, but administered separately. It also acts as a research contractor, carrying out work for the Department of Health, the Department for International Development and a number of other bodies (MRC, 2000).

Universities

Universities carry out 'in-house' research supported by the HEFCE block grant. Over and above this, universities are contractors for the other elements of the system, as well as overseas bodies. A majority of charitable funding supports research within the university sector and a substantial part of the MRC budget also supports university-based research. Like the NHS, the university sector is a provider of infrastructure, such as libraries, computing and other hardware, which other research funders exploit.

The private sector

The private for-profit sector carries out most of the research it funds in-house or through contract research organisations. These research establishments are part of the world's health research economy: most belong to international companies with R&D facilities located across the developed world. They may be moved in the light of economic and other circumstances from one country to another.

Most not-for-profit funding goes to other organisations – about 70 per cent to the university sector – but there are exceptions, e.g. the Imperial Cancer Research Fund which has in-house facilities. The AMRC website (www.amrc.org.uk) states that its members 'support a range of UK research workers, including doctors, academic scientists and research support staff'. Before its merger with the Cancer Research Campaign, the Imperial Cancer Research Fund employed over 1000 doctors and scientists carrying out over one-third of all UK cancer research.

The nature of the research economy

Although in key areas, such as the testing of drugs in clinical trials, the private sector is to some degree dependent on the NHS, its links with the NHS are relatively weak in the sense that it has its own priorities and chooses its own fields of research. The strong public interest in the location of its research and production facilities is largely explained by their contribution to the UK economy rather than their significance for the NHS.

The health research economy is a global institution. Much of the worldwide spending on health-related R&D is relevant to the NHS: drugs discovered in the USA will (usually) be available in the UK; scientific discoveries made in US laboratories are available to UK researchers and those in other countries once they have been published in the usual ways. In that part of the health research economy which is subject to the rules of commerce (the 'tradeable sector'), the UK is a competitor second only to the USA. In that part of it which is not (the 'exchange sector'), knowledge may also be exchanged through the usual process of publication in journals. The UK is also a major player in this process.

Within the tradeable sector, relevant knowledge is often concealed or, where not concealed, controlled through the use of patents. Within the exchange sector, knowledge is generally not concealed and its use not controlled. Accordingly, both international trade and international exchange contribute to the development of NHS services.

In principle, therefore, the UK health research economy could import the knowledge it requires by both of these routes. In the commercial sector it does so to some degree, either through the purchase of licences (e.g. for the manufacture of generic drugs) or through direct importation. In the non-commercial sector, where exchange is unrestricted, knowledge (e.g. the results of clinical trials) is freely imported and exported. This is not to say there are no imperfections which prevent the flow of knowledge: for example, there is strong evidence that findings of negative effects are not published as freely as those showing positive effects.

But even in principle not all the knowledge that the NHS needs can be acquired by purchase or exchange. The closer to the delivery end of health care, the more specific the required knowledge is. This specificity arises because the way that health care is actually delivered varies a great deal between countries: financing, organisation, professional roles and geography all differ between countries and to a lesser degree within them. This type of knowledge may be freely exchangeable, but not necessarily readily applicable to the local situation. Accordingly, the production of knowledge must be to some degree system-specific and most of it, as we argue in the next chapter, is not tradeable either.

Overview

This brief description of the health research economy has identified the following central features:

- It is pluralistic on both the payer and the provider side.
- The private for-profit sector is by far the largest element on both sides.
- The private not-for-profit sector contribution is larger than the Department of Health/NHS budget, but smaller than the total public sector commitment.
- The roles of the various players are interwoven: the NHS, in particular, contributes to the roles of the other players.
- The Department of Health, through the NHS, provides research infrastructure essential for the other players. The HEFCE plays the same role within universities.

■ While much of the knowledge the NHS needs is exchangeable through trade or academic exchange, much is not, but rather is peculiar to its own institutions.

In themselves these facts tell us very little. But they suggest a number of issues which later parts of this study will examine. In particular:

■ Does the UK health research economy have the best possible structure, i.e. are the balance and division of roles between its various players as effective as they might be?
■ Do the relationships between players work effectively in those areas, such as clinical research, where they are interdependent?
■ Does the UK health research economy, despite its diversity, nevertheless neglect some areas regardless of their potential to benefit patients?

Before tackling these questions, we need to consider what drives the various actors, i.e. what incentives and constraints influence the way they operate. We turn to these in the following chapter.

Chapter 2

How does the health research economy work?

The various players in the health research economy are subject to different motivations and incentives which bias their contributions. This chapter describes how these biases come about and, in this light, suggests areas in which the public sector is likely to have a critical role.

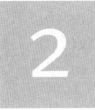

2 How does the health research economy work?

The previous chapter has demonstrated that the research economy comprises both public and private bodies with different organisational forms and embodying different incentives and constraints as funders and providers. In addition, there are strong interconnections between the players. Some providers may receive funding from all the main sources identified, while all providers must, in some circumstances, work together.

This structure has emerged: it has not been planned. At no time has the Government or any of the many committees which have considered the research economy (or, more usually, a part of it) attempted to set out what a system for the production of knowledge *should* be like.

This chapter lays some groundwork for considering how the health research economy might be improved by examining some of the fundamental assumptions upon which its current operations are based. This involves two central questions:

- What is the nature of the health research economy itself – what biases and incentives does it embody?
- How should public and private roles be determined?

This analysis leads us to identify a number of areas in the health research economy in which we would expect *only* the public sector to have a role. But we also note some inherent features of the public sector which may lead it to be inefficient or ineffective at discharging these and other roles. These findings provide the framework against which we can judge, in later chapters, how appropriately the current role of the Department of Health and other public funders has been defined and discharged.

Incentives and biases: what determines the production of health-related knowledge?[8]

The Introduction to this study set out a number of general criticisms of the health research economy. These suggest that, despite the vast volume of resources devoted to health-related research, the economy is biased against the production of certain kinds of knowledge. As a result, the aggregate of welfare produced by the NHS and the measures taken to promote health in other sectors is less than it could be. We deliberately use this vague term 'aggregate of welfare' in recognition that there is no single measure of good performance of a health care system. At this stage we are not attempting to support claims that particular areas or particular health needs are being neglected. Rather we will reflect on the systematic or underlying reasons why the health research economy may be subject to biases against certain kinds of investigation.[9]

Our approach is to uncover bias in the system, which is to say any incentives which encourage those working in the health research economy or paying for research to focus on a restricted range of areas to the neglect of others and hence, potentially, reduce the aggregate of welfare.

We do not here focus on the factors which might result in such an outcome in particular cases – the failings of individuals (e.g. scientific

---

8. See Love (2000) for a discussion which closely parallels this text. See also Spece *et al.* (1996).

9. We use the term bias here in a neutral sense. For example, in the case of the private commercial sector there is an inherent bias against non-profit-making research. If there is a bias in the public sector against some kinds of research, that may or may not be undesirable, depending on what the bias is against or in favour of. In taking this line we are consciously side-stepping the issue of what counts as 'objective'. We take it as read that no person or institution or discipline can claim to have an objective view of the world that allows a dispassionate review of the whole field of potential research areas. As will become clearer below, one of our central arguments is that the best that can be aimed for is a greater degree of democracy in the research arena to allow hitherto disfranchised areas to make their claim for resources.

See Hammersley and Gomm 1997 for a different approach to bias, which they define as 'systematic and culpable error'. We accept 'systematic' but not 'culpable', since some of the biases we believe important can be regarded as natural implications of existing economic and social institutions. However, it is clear that many do use bias to mean 'culpable'.

fraud) or active suppression of results[10] – but instead step back and look at how the system as a whole is affected by who pays for research and the incentives that that produces. We also look at how other incentives impact on what areas researchers themselves choose when they are in a position to do so.

There are a number of different points in the health research economy system where biases might arise. We take in turn the private for-profit payers, the not-for-profit sector payers, and finally the providers – the professional and other expert groups. The role of the State is discussed in relation to each of these sectors and then in its own right, summarising its role and adding a note about its own weaknesses. We use the term 'role of the State' in part as shorthand for the activities of a range of Government departments and public bodies and in part to abstract from the specifics of current policy so as to focus on what the *general* justifications are for public action in the area we are examining. At this stage we are not attempting to assess what the Department of Health is doing now.

Payers: for-profit companies and market failure

We have seen how private pharmaceutical companies, to which may be added non-pharmaceutical companies producing, for example, surgical equipment or diagnostic techniques, are by far the biggest spenders on research. They rely ultimately on the NHS (as well as exports to the health care systems of other countries) and thus indirectly on the State for the bulk of their income.

The incentives at work in these companies are clearly associated with the principal motor of private sector activity – the profit motive. Thus the

---

10. See Martin (1999) for a substantial review of the failures in the research economy which can be attributed to practices which fall short of the assumed norm of openness in science. He states that: 'In spite of rhetoric of openness in research, the practice is often quite different. There are numerous examples of suppression, including pressures not to undertake research in the first place, institutional controls on dissemination of data, and attacks on researchers who produce unwelcome results. A few types of suppression are severely stigmatised, such as research fraud that has the effect of distorting or submerging accurate data. Other types of suppression do not evoke universal condemnation, but may generate concern on a case-by-case basis, such as the use of defamation law to prevent publication. Finally, there are some types of suppression that are commonplace and widely accepted, such as secrecy of research undertaken under the aegis of national security' (Martin, 1999, p.2).

principal, if not the only, reason for them to become involved in research is to develop products which will contribute to future revenues and shareholder value. In this respect, they are no different from any other industry supplying services which the NHS needs. Pharmaceutical companies are simply the most extreme example of firms which must invest and develop their product range through the generation of new knowledge.

Disincentives caused by knowledge as a public good

The problem with new knowledge as an economic commodity is that it is difficult to retain for the use of the company that produces it. Any innovative product or service can be copied by other firms which did not contribute to the cost of investing in the research necessary for the innovation. In fact it is difficult to think of goods and services which do not suffer from this problem in their product development phase, and almost impossible to think of a good where at least the production process itself might not benefit from research and innovation, if only to make it more efficient. If such innovations become freely available once a product is on the market, allowing others a 'free ride', there is a built-in disincentive for firms to spend on producing the knowledge underlying innovations which can easily be copied.

Such new knowledge has some of the characteristics of what economists call 'public goods', both those for which it is impossible to provide some benefit (or impose a cost) without simultaneously doing so for everyone: indivisibility; and those where one person's consumption does not impinge on the ability of others to consume: non-rivalness (Barr, 1998). In the extreme case, knowledge of this kind is available to everyone or no one. Less extremely, there are 'externalities': the benefit to the knowledge producer also provides benefits to many other people who did not contribute to the cost of producing it.

While an 'idea' is not expensive to pass on once it has come into existence, getting the idea in the first place can be very expensive. If this effort is discouraged because the developer of a new idea cannot derive sufficient profit from it, then this might not be in the best interest of the consumer, because research could be stifled before it gets off the ground.

In economic terms this constitutes a classic trade-off between static and dynamic efficiency (Lazear, 1999). Static efficiency requires that at any given point in time goods are supplied at marginal cost – very low for most knowledge-type goods. Dynamic efficiency requires that incentives (profits) are sufficient to promote the research in the first place so that benefits accrue subsequently over a period of time.

Patent protection

The most common resolution of this tension has been to offer a compromise: the patent. This enables a company to have sole rights to exploit a particular innovation for a period of time, thus allowing profits to be generated. (In economic terms, the legal rule provides for the 'internalisation' of the external benefits.) However, after this time period is up, the use of the new knowledge becomes available to all and competition should ensure that marginal-cost pricing results. The length of the patent is intended to balance the need to provide incentives for R&D with the desire to minimise the cost of products to the consumer.

The tension between the need to provide incentives and the need to extend the benefits of the results is particularly acute in the health research economy. There are enormous research and regulatory approval costs and unusually high degrees of uncertainty in bringing products to market. Most important, the final products can be imitated at low cost (Long, 1999). Once a new drug comes on to the market, other firms can analyse its chemical make-up and simply reproduce it, competing away all the economic advantage. The risks attached to commercial investment in R&D are, therefore, enormous.[11] Most privately funded research therefore would not take place without the protection offered by patents.

This protection is not, however, sufficient in itself to ensure that the private sector carries out all the R&D that the NHS may require. There are a number of areas in which the incentives for the private sector may be insufficient to motivate research.

---

11. Patents are generally granted only for products which are new, useful and non-obvious. This is taken to include anything made by humankind and therefore excludes discoveries – things which are already in existence, such as human genes, but not previously discovered. However, DNA sequences and genetically modified organisms may be patented because these are altered or purified versions of naturally occurring things. See Sulston and Ferry (2002) for an insider view of where the dividing line between patentable and non-patentable has been and should be drawn.

Short-termism

First, the for-profit sector is often criticised for being short-termist. For example, Drews, an industry insider, writes: '[Businesspeople] do not readily get involved with a research strategy with uncertain outcome that, even if it were not very expensive, nonetheless consumes a great deal of time.' (Drews, 1998, p.185). This short-termism is blamed on institutional shareholders constantly requiring increased dividends. Such pressure can lead companies to seek relatively quick and predictable profits, and thus research strategies which promise returns in the short run, rather than those with more distant and less certain outcomes. This may be reflected in a reluctance to investigate the mechanisms underlying diseases.

For example, delving into the mysteries of the operation of cells at a basic level may not directly produce any specific outcome beneficial to health, but may produce immensely influential and important discoveries with widespread beneficial applications in the future. However, the process may be too slow for shareholders seeking a competitive return on their investment.

Seeking large potential markets

Second, the for-profit sector will seek to pursue research which has the expectation of producing the largest potential profit and thus will tend to be directed towards those states of ill health which affect the largest numbers of people. This tendency is exacerbated by the growth of very large drug companies, itself in part fuelled by risk avoidance – much of that risk arising from the regulatory process.

In itself, this is no bad thing: cures for cancer, for example, or for less serious but common complaints such as flu or stomach ulcers are clearly desirable. But if this is the only driving force for research, certain categories of person – in particular those with rare forms of disease – might be excluded from the pursuit of new cures altogether. Equally, as the arguments about the availability of AIDS drugs in developing countries indicate, certain diseases may be neglected because those suffering from them and their governments do not have the purchasing power to attract investment in their cure, prevention or relief.

As the availability of patents indicates, however, what the private sector will have an incentive to do depends on the framework within which it operates. The State may wish to ensure that every category of patient, no matter how small numerically, is offered the prospect of some chance of innovative treatments being discovered. Here a special variant of patient protection or other incentives may be offered to induce supply. The USA, for example, has an Orphan Drugs Act to overcome this problem (see, for example, Haffner, 1998; Shulman and Manocchia, 1997; Thamer *et al.*, 1998; Minghetti *et al.*, 2000). In the UK and the rest of Europe related regimes exist – not that the mere existence of such regimes implies that they are adequate.

Disincentives to research in the social science field

There is a third area where the private sector may not be a willing investor in the acquisition of new knowledge – often knowledge in the social science field – where the subject matter is the operation of the public service itself. There is little incentive for the private sector to *pay* for social science research, whether into the delivery of care, the ethics or public accountability of the service or the wider political and sociological context of the service (although many private consultants will readily investigate existing knowledge bases and *provide* this knowledge for the State in return for a fee). The market for such knowledge is limited, in the case of the NHS, to a single purchaser.

There are, of course, areas such as management techniques and software which rely to some degree on R&D, but the risks involved are much less than in drug development and there are, typically, alternative markets for such services outside the NHS itself. In general, however, we would not expect that the private sector would make major investments in R&D bearing primarily on service delivery and the broader context in which the NHS operates.

Similarly the NHS (or the public sector) requires knowledge relating to certain types of public health measure and to epidemiological research into the factors in the economic, social and physical environment that give rise to disease or encourage its spread, or those which tend to promote good health. The knowledge required to implement measures designed to tackle the causes of ill health cannot be sold over and over again to a buyer – once a successful public health measure has been developed it is effectively unpatentable. Knowledge of the impact on health of poor housing or lack of social support, or that certain forms of diet or exercise are beneficial, is unlikely to be marketable (although some public health technologies, such as nicotine replacement patches, are exceptions).

The regulatory regime and research into negative impacts of products

The private sector has only a limited incentive to search for the negative impact on health of products within and outside the health field unless the regulatory regime specifically requires it to do so. However, the incentives to produce such knowledge depend, as do the incentives to research into new drugs to cure disease, on the prevailing legal and regulatory framework. The most important of these is the regime for approving the introduction of new treatments – in particular the nature of the evidence required before they are accepted for use within the NHS. From the private sector viewpoint, the approval regime has become increasingly onerous, particularly with the introduction of NICE which has added additional tests (in particular cost-effectiveness) to those imposed by the Medicines Control Agency and its European counterparts.

Recent NICE assessments, for example its evaluation of beta interferon, have brought out how incomplete the evidence relating to the impact of new drugs often is, precisely because existing arrangements do not compel its collection. In principle, the approval regime could do so by, for example, combining the role of the Medicines Control Agency and NICE[12] and making it impossible to gain approval for general use before a range of potential risks have been evaluated.[13] Equally, other arrangements can be envisaged to encourage the development of new drugs or treatments, such as competitions which promise a large reward to those who are successful (see Kremer, 1998 for a discussion of other options).

Finally, the nature of the compensation regimes available to individuals who claim to have suffered damage from drugs may be critical. The more rigorous they are, the greater the incentives for companies to test thoroughly for undesirable side-effects (see, for example, Mundy, 2001) and the greater the risks inherent in bringing a drug to market.[14]

To sum up: the overall motivation of the private sector is clear enough. How that plays out in practice is in some measure determined by the

---

12. There are practical arguments against such a merger (see Cowper, 2001).

13. In the case of beta interferon the Department of Health came to an agreement with the industry which meant that it would pay only when the drug was successful – the first time such an arrangement had been made.

14. We are not advocating such changes here, but simply making the point that the incentives for the private sector can be set in a range of ways.

precise legal and regulatory framework within which it operates. The use of patents and controls over safety are virtually universal regulatory features of the world health economy. Both leave the initiative with the private sector as to what areas to invest research resources in. As we shall see later, other forms of relationship are feasible.

Payers: the voluntary sector and 'charitable failure'

Chapter 1 showed that the not-for-profit sector is a surprisingly significant player in the provision of resources for medical research, with the top six charitable spenders contributing almost as much as the entire NHS R&D programme. The motives driving the for-profit sector are clear enough, and the circumstances in which markets may fail and the State have a role are well understood. But how should we think about the role of the voluntary sector?[15]

Defining 'the voluntary sector'

As a preliminary, it is worth outlining the elements of a definition of the voluntary sector. Forming a definition is by no means straightforward, but Kendall and Knapp (1996) report that the international consensus was that only bodies which meet all four of the following criteria should be considered voluntary:

- formal – having structured constitutions or formal sets of rules
- independent of Government and self-governing – not directly controlled by for-profit or State enterprises and with their own internal decision-making structures
- non-profit-distributing and primarily non-business – thus excluding 'mutual' organisations such as building societies and motoring organisations, even if they have no shareholders as such
- 'voluntary' – there should be an element of voluntarism, either in donation of money or labour, including wages at less than market rates, or unpaid service on governing boards.

---

15. In this chapter, the voluntary, charitable and not-for-profit sectors are treated as synonymous. The literature on the voluntary sector in this context is not well developed. Although much has been written about the voluntary sector, the modern social science disciplines have tended to relegate discussion of its role in modern society to that of a side-show to the main event of the 'state v. market' debate. More recently, however, theoretical discussions of its potential role as a provider of welfare and other services have re-emerged.

Most medical charities satisfy most or all of these criteria and indeed score heavily in the final criterion through the large sums of money received and given away in grants for research.

Reasons for voluntary sector involvement

Why is there a need for a charitable sector within the health research economy? Is there a rationale for its existence beyond simply the manifestation of the spontaneous desire of particular groups of people to promote some or other good – in the present context, better treatment for a particular disease group.[16] It is this notion which probably forms the 'common-sense' understanding of many charitable organisations, particularly those which are involved with giving in cash or kind. Humane and compassionate people see others in need, or see some public issue which needs promoting, and band together to raise money or offer their time. Medical charities typically grow up around such perceptions of specific illnesses and many of those involved will have close experience of the disease and simply wish to do something about it, even if they themselves do not directly benefit.

One implication of the creation of such organisations is that, in the eyes of the members of these bodies, the State does not do enough. In other words, we might look to the State to operate in the areas in which the commercial private sector is unwilling to invest, but the State itself may 'fail', i.e. its priorities and its perceptions of 'the needs of the NHS' may not coincide with those of some individuals.

One might think, therefore, that the activities of these bodies are unproblematic, possibly without further analytical interest. In a liberal democracy people are allowed to engage in any sort of legal activity as long as they do no harm, and giving money to scientists to conduct research is just one such activity. Indeed, the State goes some way to assisting these activities by providing tax breaks and other financial help to bodies with charitable status. But this in itself raises the question of why such help should be forthcoming – if a tax break can be given, why should the State not spend this money itself?

One answer appears to lie in the special role the voluntary sector plays in society, by undertaking economic and political activities which would be

---

16. Most medical charities fall into this category – see list of AMRC members at www.amrc.org.uk.

difficult if not impossible under other forms of organisation. The various theories which contribute to this explanation are either economic in their focus, concerned with the sector's potential for improving aggregate welfare, or political/sociological, concerned with why the sector exists and with its relationship with the State.[17] It is impossible to do justice to the wide range of theoretical perspectives on the voluntary sector, and here we simply pick out three of the most significant.

Filling gaps

The first perspective builds on the standard rationale for State involvement where there are (quasi-) public goods (Weisbrod, 1977). The State must make a collective decision on how much research to finance. But it is almost certain that the level decided upon will fall short of the wishes of some voters and exceed those of others relative to their tax contributions. There will be some who consider the level decided upon as an 'under-supply'. If so, there is scope for them to correct such a 'Government failure' by contributing to charitable foundations which then augment the aggregate national spend on research.

Of course, the free-rider problem has not gone away: those who do not contribute will nevertheless benefit from the (additional) research. But those who view State provision as too low may have no alternative but to 'swallow' the free-rider problem and accept that the fruits of their contribution will be enjoyed by everyone – indeed by the very nature of the voluntary sector they may be content to accept this.

Lack of trust in other funders of research

The second major theoretical perspective – the contract failure theory – also starts from an analysis of the market and its failures (Hansmann, 1980). When we wish to give to others we may simply not trust for-profit companies to do as honourable a job as the not-for-profit sector – even if the profit motive makes commercial organisations more efficient at doing so and more than compensates for the need to distribute dividends. More simply, profit-making may simply *seem* inappropriate when altruistic giving is concerned – indeed it is just about impossible to think of any for-profit firms engaged purely in altruistic activity. Here, it

---

17. We are not concerned here with the role of pressure groups (although many of the voluntary bodies mentioned do undertake this role as well), but with the political/economic functions of welfare service providers or funders – in the case of knowledge generation, chiefly the latter.

is the non-distribution criterion that is critical, because 'consumers' of an agency's activities are more likely to believe that the agency genuinely holds their interests at heart, and is not trying in some way to take advantage of a situation, if that agency is not proposing to distribute profits.

This may be particularly true where vulnerable people are concerned or where the product is a very complex one, as in health care research. Such a role for the not-for-profit sector can thus be reassuring to individuals. It can also be efficient from a societal viewpoint because otherwise rather more resources would need to be devoted to monitoring and regulation of for-profit firms and there would be leakage of resources to shareholders' dividends (this does not imply that voluntary sector agencies are necessarily more efficient, as we will see).

Again, one may ask why the voluntary sector should be necessary rather than the State which, after all, is not driven by the profit motive either. But the State may also be bedevilled by lack of trust, not least that taxes actually go towards uses that the voters really value. While public pressure may be exerted for some such neglected areas, voluntary agencies focused on small disease groups are unlikely to have such political muscle. In these circumstances, perhaps *only* the voluntary sector can really reassure people that their financial contribution is used for the ends they desire.

Acting as a 'buffer zone'

Third, and from a more political/sociological perspective, is a set of theories that emphasise the voluntary sector acting as a kind of 'buffer zone' between State and society. In this account, the sector acts as a kind of 'shunting yard' for unsolvable social problems. Here it is not any perceived advantage in terms of social efficiency that underpins its existence, but its ability to give the impression that 'something is being done' about issues that are inherently intractable. It should be said that this is usually in the guise of a service provider rather than funder, but some medical charities may provide such a service even when they simply act as funders.

Other perspectives

Other theoretical perspectives emphasise the partnership and mutual dependency between the State and voluntary sectors, rather than a simplistic competitive model emphasising which is the 'right' sector to provide services or finance. Rather than the voluntary sector being a gap-filler in response to failures in other sectors, the State and voluntary sector have in fact developed in co-operation. In short, during the growth of the welfare state, the State and non-profit sectors have tended to develop in ways which play to each other's strengths and mitigate each other's weaknesses.

To sum up: where the State cannot provide public goods such as research in adequate quantities or where it is not trusted to make wise decisions in fields open to private action, the voluntary sector has a role.

Weaknesses of the voluntary sector

The voluntary sector also has its weaknesses, which provide the State with its continuing and complementary role. These carry the unattractive labels of insufficiency, particularism, paternalism and amateurism.

Insufficiency mirrors the State's inability to deal sufficiently with the welfare needs of the citizens in advanced societies. In the voluntary sector's case the difficulty is in generating enough resources through voluntary donation or other income-generating schemes, and ensuring that these resources are reliably available over time. The State, on the other hand, has the ability to tax and generate a (generally) reliable income stream.

Particularism reflects the voluntary sector's concern with particular client groups, which may conflict with equity. Equity requires a strategic approach, and only one concept of the proper distribution of benefits and burdens in society can be applied at any point in time. A reasoned view of how benefits should be distributed between groups cannot simply be the aggregate of what individual voluntary groups are able to obtain – not least because some will be more powerful and wealthier than others. In a pluralist society this variation in size and influence of voluntary groups will inevitably prevail, but it should not seduce us into thinking that what emerges is necessarily fair. The State, as the only democratic institution and the only one with the legal ability to coerce, may wish to counteract the results of this 'natural' process to promote what it considers a more equitable outcome.

Paternalism reflects the fact that since much voluntary sector activity is dependent on financial donations or volunteer labour, such donations tend to come from the higher-income sectors of society. People who donate money, or their labour time, wish to exercise some kind of control over how these resources are used. Thus there is a tendency for the objectives of the voluntary sector to reflect the perceptions, goals and attitudes of the relatively well-off. The point is that even if these goals and attitudes are well intentioned and focused on the needs of the needy, they may reflect only a partial understanding of the proper response to those needs, and in particular not take proper account of what the recipients themselves wish.[18]

Amateurism has also been a criticism of the charitable sector since the 19th century, reflecting some of the problems associated with paternalism. The growth of the welfare state led to calls for the professionalisation of welfare services and accordingly a limit to the scope of voluntary agencies that could often afford only the well-meaning amateur. To some extent this problem remains, with trustees of voluntary organisation often being well-intentioned individuals with sufficient resources to allow them to give their time freely to promote some non-profitable purpose, but without necessarily having formal training or having studied the problem in any rigorous way.

These four criticisms may, however, have less force in respect of the voluntary role in health-related research than in other areas: the needs of someone suffering from a rare disease are largely independent of their economic and social circumstances (though these may affect its incidence and impact). Furthermore, what we have identified as potential weaknesses may in fact represent the greatest strengths of voluntary action. Those moved to support it often have close experience of the diseases in question and the organisations themselves may in some areas be more professional than the professionals. Besides, most health charities call on the advice of experienced professionals in their field.

Nevertheless, our analysis suggests that the State may have to play a 'corrective' role to the voluntary sector, just as the voluntary sector may fill the 'gaps' left by the public and private sectors. In other words, while the private sector may be relied on to work in certain ways because

---

18. This paternalistic tendency has always been a bugbear of the charitable sector, ever since the 19th-century philanthropic attitude that the poor were essentially responsible for their own destitution, and that the wealthier classes had a responsibility to lift them up and educate them out of their profligate ways. Paternalism in the 21st century is doubtless less overt, but the critique remains. The State, of course, is also seen as paternalistic, but its advantage is that there are formal lines of democratic accountability open to all sectors of the community and not just to those who contribute (the highest) taxes.

its incentives are clear, this is less true of the voluntary sector. It is inherently less predictable in terms of what it will do and how well it will do it.

Providers: scientific researchers and the professions

So far we have concentrated our analysis on how new knowledge production is financed, and the incentives and biases inherent in the institutional means by which this occurs. But there are those who actually conduct the research: the scientists, academic researchers and members of professions who also spend part of their time undertaking original research. These individuals will certainly be influenced by the decisions of funders, and therefore by their incentives and biases, for the simple reason that the granting of research monies will often be accompanied by some kind of specification of the research to be undertaken. And of course those working within or for the private sector have to accept the nature of the incentives which drive the sector.

In recent years, parts of the public sector, particularly the universities, have been encouraged to adopt some incentives normally associated with the private sector by turning intellectual capital which in the past may have been a public good into private goods to the financial benefit of both the individuals and the institutions concerned. (In January 2002 the Secretary of State for Health announced proposals to encourage NHS trusts to do the same.) Similarly, the way in which universities function within the health research economy may be influenced by the extent of private funding and other forms of interaction between commerce and academe.[19]

Nevertheless, academic scientists often have a significant degree of freedom to establish their own research priorities, academic medics do 'own account' research and many voluntary foundations – such as the King's Fund itself – will employ researchers who are then allowed a degree of latitude in pursuing their own research interests. The same is true of some private sector research establishments. And even programmes of research which are more carefully specified by the funders

---

19. We allude here to a large subject which we do not aim to cover, i.e. the 'corruption' of apparently independent institutions and individuals by profit-seeking behaviour. We look at this issue briefly in Chapter 8.

will often allow the researcher the opportunity to influence the research to reflect priorities other than those of the funder.

Furthermore, in whichever part of the health research economy researchers are located, they will tend to be influenced by generally prevailing views as to which areas are worth researching and what methods to use.[20] As a result, bias may enter into the work of apparently independent researchers. Here we consider three sources of such bias: the conformity to certain orthodoxies and research norms, various forms of self-interest and intellectual curiosity. We do not consider here conflicts of interest where researchers or others have financial interests in the outcomes of their own work. This issue has generated a massive literature (see Resnik, 1999).

Conformity to norms

To become a scientist, or any dedicated professional researcher, one must undergo prolonged training. During this time, it is argued, prospective scientists tend to accept the values, standards and assumptions of science as presented by previous generations. Non-conformists are not encouraged because of the need to pass exams. The outcome is that originality or radically new ideas are unlikely to develop. Essentially the argument is that educational communities are rather inflexible and conservative, and have a bias towards the way things have been understood in the past.

Adding to this rigidity is what Martin calls 'the social system of science':

> *after a long period of training and socialisation, a scientist begins to practise science as part of the scientific community. The scientist practises science in a social system – a set of relationships between people and an established set of practices and patterns of behaviour.*

> Martin, 1979, p.63[21]

The central element in this social system is various forms of peer pressure. Researchers depend on their colleagues for approval of their research. They may have greater access to jobs, research facilities and

20. The literature is vast, but the classic work is Kuhn (1962).

21. In another paper Martin (1999) systematically assesses the process by which research data are suppressed.

research grants depending on how they are viewed by their (typically 'senior') colleagues. In this process, innovative ideas may be squeezed out: to gain acceptance, research must be carried out in particular areas in particular ways.

In medicine perhaps the most interesting example here is the development of the randomised control trial (RCT) and more generally of evidence-based medicine. At first this was strongly resisted by the medical profession as offending notions of clinical freedom: it required clinicians to adopt standardised methodologies rather than applying their own individual judgement. It was this latter principle which had become embedded in medical norms over hundreds of years.

Gradually the notion that statistical methodologies and – even more slowly – costs and benefits should be taken into account gained ground, but only because of the efforts of rival groups of experts such as economists and statisticians alongside a small group of maverick clinicians. But now, ironically, the growing hegemony of the RCT and 'gold-standard' trials is liable to be criticised from outside the 'new' orthodoxy, with claims that any innovation that cannot readily submit itself to a RCT is being neglected regardless of the strength of other kinds of evidence.[22]

In all these ways, tightly 'organized, self-reflective groups of specialists who pursue communal goals' (Lowrance, 1985) serve to reinforce the *status quo* and inhibit the introduction of new, radical ideas that might upset existing hierarchies and power relations. Furthermore, attempts to ensure that research monies are well spent through the process of peer review tend to reinforce this tendency. In particular, Horrobin, argues that:

> *peer review, as at present practised threatens progress in clinical medicine. Peer review fails to promote innovation, either in clinical or*

---

22. One such case which has been subjected to an in-depth review in this context is acupuncture (Saks, 1995). The conclusion of the study is that the power of the medical profession, and its self-interest, has served to exclude acupuncture from standard medical practice. Saks essentially sees self-interest in terms of wealth, power and prestige (of which more below) and argues that it may be in the interests of the profession to seek to exclude 'alternative' medicine from professional recognition because to admit it will weaken the position of its members who have no expertise in these procedures, and thus fear that their ability to continue to accrue rewards will wane. The point here, however, is that one orthodoxy can replace another and can introduce a new sort of bias into the system, even if one believes it to be an improvement on previous practice.

basic research. ... Diversity – which is essential, since experts cannot know the source of the next major discovery – is not encouraged

Horrobin, 1996, p.1294[23]

Although peer review is still the norm in prestigious journals, even its practitioners are sceptical of its value (see, for example, Smith, 1999). However, Horrobin's very severe strictures have not been widely accepted. But Baum (2002) argues that peer review (combined with developments in cancer research funding) are posing threats to diversity in the field of cancer research.

Self-interest

The second theme which emerges from the literature is linked to the first – that of self-interest (Martin, 1979; Jevons, 1973). This may simply be reflected in the desire of researchers to be awarded the honours and prestige which comes from doing work recognised by their peers as excellent – and which may also have a tendency to conservatism as a result. Proctor, for example writes:

A cancer cured is tangible, a marvellous success, but a cancer prevented is invisible, a statistical abstraction. Prizes abound for cancer cures, but where are the prizes for cancer prevention?

Proctor, 1995, p.268

But self-interest can also manifest itself in the constant demands of the research community that 'further research is necessary', thereby evading the need to suggest policy answers in favour of continually reformulating and refining the question. Such a motivation can also lead to the exaggeration of claims about the importance of research, a charge which is sometimes made against those currently promoting the importance of genome research (see, for example, Jones, 2000). The more scientists

---

23. Horrobin has been one of the fiercest critics of peer review, arguing that it tends to promote conformity or worse: 'I suspect that peer reviewers sometimes subconsciously give hard reviews to clinical projects, ostensibly because the science is poor, but in reality because they fear successful outcomes – the advent of cures would herald the demise of most research funds in their field. I am not suggesting that the "policy" is deliberate and iniquitous in intent. I contend that the decisions are indubitably harsh, and the consequences flowing from them are as devastating to clinical investigators as if they were the intended victims of crime. I am aware of five detailed case histories – two related to muscular dystrophy, two to multiple sclerosis, and one to schizophrenia – in which the rejection of clinical research programmes was, in my view, explicable only on this basis' (Horrobin, 1996, p.1294).

hype the potential of such research, the more likely they are to create a climate in which that research is supported financially – even if the tangible applications remain limited. Personal honours are also behind the desire for many scientists to be 'first', another potential bias in encouraging the exaggeration or manipulation of findings.

Intellectual curiosity

Finally, the role of intellectual curiosity, or the 'pleasure of research' (Jevons, 1973). It has often been mentioned in the literature on rationing or priority-setting in the NHS that one potentially inappropriate consideration for a consultant when deciding whom next to admit from a waiting list is to consider the clinically 'interesting' case (New, 1996). Behind this concern is the idea that one incentive for scientists and researchers is the intellectual satisfaction of doing the work. This may lead to exciting new discoveries – but these may not lead quickly to innovations capable of improving health or, if they do, they do so only in a very indirect way and not in proportion to the resources devoted to the original research.

As Jevons (1973) puts it: 'What many people find startling ... is the assertion that hardly any industrial processes are based on discoveries made in curiosity-oriented science.' By this he means that 'technology' (industrial processes) usually arises from specific targeted attempts to improve matters. Pure research does not directly contribute to useful knowledge.

In health care this is less of a danger – even the most 'pure' biological research does at least in principle have a focus – that of improving health. But the point is worth making that what can be intellectually stimulating – such as the development of knowledge about the human genome – *may* not lead to outcomes of benefit to people, or to outcomes in proportion to the resources put in. Less intellectually stimulating research – such as developing better joint replacements or devices for tackling incontinence – may be of the most benefit, but may be perceived as 'boring' and certainly not likely to qualify the researcher for any of science's glittering prizes.

But while this analysis suggests that 'research is too important to be left to the researchers', it is equally obvious that to a large degree it must be, for only those with specialist knowledge or experience can actually envisage what might be done and then do it. It follows that at the heart of the health research economy is the thorny issue of how, if at all, those who are ultimately the customers for its products, can have a say, as they do in other markets, as to what those products should be.

The role of the State

Our analysis suggests that there are several areas where the State may be required to fill in potential gaps in the health research economy:

- It can support long-term science and 'pure' science. This is broadly the role of the MRC (and to a less extent the other research councils) and the higher education funding councils.
- It can support research where small potential aggregate benefits are justified on equity grounds, particularly when the voluntary sector does not fill the gap and where the work required is at the applied end of the spectrum, i.e. is of little scientific interest.
- It can produce knowledge bearing on the running the NHS, including the role of politicians, managers and clinicians. This is the area we refer to as 'the needs of the NHS'. It includes research in support of public health measures.
- It can fill other gaps in the activities of both parts of the private sector. This might involve offering financial support or other encouragement to the private sector to engage in new areas of research or product development where risks are high. The Medlink programme and some elements of the work of the Department of Trade and Industry come into this category.

But the State also has potential weaknesses, some of which were mentioned during our discussion of the voluntary sector. The principal ones for our purposes are summarised usefully in Le Grand (1991). Briefly:

- The State may act like a monopoly, particularly where it is captured by particular sets of views as to what kind of research to carry out and what areas to research into or when the State itself takes a strong evidence-based position and may as a result be unwilling to fund research which could undermine it. So, while in principle it may be a 'gap filler', in practice it may be subject to the same kind of limitations as other parts of the health research economy.
- Where the State pays for research there is the problem of knowing what the proper level of funding is and how it should be determined. Like spending on health itself, there is no obvious technical method for deciding how much should be spent.

If in practice officials and experts are delegated to decide on the level of spending, they may act as budget maximisers, artificially inflating the importance of their work. In other words, some of the supply-side incentives operating in the private sector may also act in the public.

The State has other roles which may affect the way the private parts of the health research economy works, principally through the terms of patent law, drug and device licensing and compensation arrangements for those suffering from the side-effects of drugs, as well as the tax regime applicable to charities. It may also have the role, currently addressed in England and Wales through NICE, of acting as monopsony buyer of new technologies (including medicines) and promoting 'best practice' among professionals and in this way safeguard the interests of 'ill-informed' users.[24] These roles are not our concern in this study, but the way in which they are carried out may well have an impact on the readiness of the private sector to commit funds to health-related research.

Finally, the State may also work *with* the private sector in financial partnership where projects would not otherwise go ahead. We consider this role in Chapter 6.

Overview

The analytic view of the health research economy developed here reflects the 'real' economy described in Chapter 1. It is pluralistic not only in its institutions, but also in respect of the incentives and disincentives which drive it. These incentives and disincentives are not necessarily immutable. The State may modify the way the private sector works and also the way its own institutions function.

---

24. It is conventional in health care studies to assume an asymmetry of information as between professionals and users, which in turn implies a need to regulate health care provision, e.g. by controlling entry through licensing either by professional self or state regulation. This assumption is being undermined, as we see in Chapter 8, by a number of factors, not least the increasing availability of knowledge via the Internet and other sources. The asymmetry assumption would also seem to apply to research since most users are not possessors of specialist knowledge of science and of potentially fruitful areas of research. To the extent that this is true, the State may act as an agent for the user in the same way as does the clinician both in choosing areas for research and taking measures to ensure its quality. However, as we shall see below, this argument is also declining in significance.

Whatever incentives and constraints are in place, the role of any one part of the health research economy depends to a degree on what the other parts do and how they operate. Some forms of research require the participation of more than one player and also of players outside the research economy itself. We look further at these issues in Chapter 6.

The role of the public sector is itself diverse, acting as regulator, customer, provider and payer. As far as the last of these roles is concerned, the framework we have adopted leads to the conclusion that the payer role can be seen as 'gap filler', to be targeted on those areas which the other parts of the health research economy do not cover.

In the next part of this study we focus on how the payer role has been discharged within the public sector.

Chapter 3

Policy development: research funded by the Department of Health

In 1988 the House of Lords Select Committee on Science and Technology identified a series of failings in the management and organisation of medical research. Since then the Department of Health has made sustained attempts to overcome the weaknesses identified. This chapter examines policy developments in the system for financing health research, which falls within the ambit of the Department of Health and the NHS.

3 Policy development: research funded by the Department of Health

In this and the following two chapters, we focus on that part of publicly financed R&D which falls within the ambit of the Department of Health. For the last ten years, the Department has consistently attempted to manage and direct the funds at its disposal, including those deployed within the NHS, so as to increase their contribution to the 'aggregate of welfare' produced by health-preserving and health-promoting activities. In other words, it has attempted to ensure that the funds make the greatest possible contribution to 'the health of the nation'. The central question is whether these efforts have resulted in any improvement in the allocation of resources or in the overall arrangements for their management.

We begin with finance, since changes to the way that R&D is funded have been and remain central to the management of the programme as a whole: without effective financial control, other tasks, particularly implementing any centrally determined priorities, would be impossible to discharge. At its most basic level, this requires that decision makers should be able to identify the level of resources currently deployed and be able to influence the distribution of those resources. This requirement may seem too obvious to be worth stating – but in fact the present Government persists in 'allocating' funds to areas such as cancer care without the means to track whether they are used as intended.

This chapter looks at changes over recent decades in the system for funding publicly financed health R&D and at the shortcomings in information systems which have bedevilled attempts to decide how to allocate such funding.

Beginnings

The first commitment of public funds to health research occurred in 1913 with the establishment of the Medical Research Committee, later the Medical Research Council. The National Health Service Act (1946) gave the Minister of Health powers to 'conduct research or assist by grants … research into any matters relating to the causation, prevention, diagnosis of illness or mental defectiveness'. For some time, however, the Ministry of Health confined its research programme to public health. It was not until the 1960s that it formulated a research programme in all the areas allowed by the Act. By 1958 the Chief Medical Officer had a small research fund at his disposal. Four years later a departmental section concerned with research had been created and by 1967 there was a departmental research committee administering a budget of £750,000 (see McLachlan, 1971 and 1978, for more details).

In 1971, Lord Rothschild reported on R&D across the whole of Government (Rothschild, 1971). The central idea underlying his recommendations was the need to introduce a customer/provider relationship so as to improve the alignment between the work of Government research establishments and the needs of Government departments. The subsequent white paper (Cabinet Office, 1972), led to a quarter of the MRC's budget being transferred from the science vote to the health vote, roughly the proportion of the MRC's budget that was estimated to be spent on applied research. It was thought that a customer department might be able to exercise control over this 25 per cent, leaving the remaining 75 per cent to be provider-driven.

The Rothschild proposals, however, were not aimed simply at exercising some degree of control over an otherwise autonomous agency: they were also intended to create a more informed purchaser of research. In the event, the budget transfer achieved very little – the 'informed purchaser' did not emerge – and in 1981 the transfer was reversed.[25] In its place a concordat was reached between the MRC and the Department which set out in general terms the roles and interests of the two parties (see Chapter 6).

---

25. McLachlan (1978, pp.35–36), however, says that the changes 'gave a jolt of realism to Medical Research Council discussions. The relevance of proposed research programmes in terms of social need became important factors at all levels of Council deliberations.'

During the 1970s attempts were made to foster research activity in the Department of Health and Social Security. A chief scientist was appointed in 1972 to set up an organisation for commissioning research within it (see Introduction to McLachlan, 1978). In the second half of the decade a series of research liaison groups were established. These represented a development of the notion of the Department as the research customer, encouraging as they did interchange between policy makers (i.e. civil servants) and researchers. Some prospered but others did not (McLachlan, 1978, p.46).

From as early as 1958, there had been a locally organised research scheme. This absorbed some 8 per cent of the Department of Health and Social Security research budget in 1975/76, but there was no requirement that the work funded reflected national or regional priorities. Nor was there any attempt to assess whether the work was worthwhile after the event.

In 1978 the Nuffield Provincial Hospitals Trust (now the Nuffield Trust) published the report of a working party, which concluded that the Department 'has seemed to be lacking a definable research policy on which judgement can be formed by external critics' (McLachlan, 1978, p.67). It went on to raise the central issue bearing on the role of research funded by the Department, asking how the present system could possibly have an overview of the health system generally (McLachlan, 1978, p.73).

With that analysis in mind it concluded that:

> *... in order to achieve the necessary direction and control there is a case for there to be an overall body concerned with the health system as a whole, rather than a range of individual customers or client groups.*

> McLachlan, 1978, p.83

This observation received no policy response. A further Nuffield report, published in 1984, found that: 'The problem remains very much the same, indeed in sharpened form' (McLachlan, 1985, p.4). It goes on: 'The importance of identifying the elements of a *well-integrated system* for the functions of intelligence gathering, commissioning and funding in the realm of health service research is still not clearly understood.'

Nevertheless, some progress appears to have been made during this period. In his foreword to the 1990 (and last) edition of the Department of Health's annual report on its R&D programme, Francis O'Grady, the last departmental chief scientist, stated that the locally organised research scheme:

> is generally acknowledged [to have] succeeded in encouraging many who might not otherwise have done so to engage in research. ... [but] ... Many needs and opportunities are waiting to be exploited.
>
> Department of Health, 1990, p.4

By the time that the 1990 report was published, however, change was already under way.

Policy since 1988

The 1988 House of Lords report

The main turning point in the development of policy towards R&D funded by the Department of Health and Social Security was the report into medical research of the Science and Technology Committee of the House of Lords, published in 1988 (and referred to below as the 1988 report).[26] Despite its focus on medicine, the 1988 report ranged very widely and we draw on it extensively in this and following chapters.

Against the background set out above, it is no surprise that the 1988 report identified a series of failings in the organisation and management of medical research. Assessing the overall position, it concluded that:

> The Chief Scientist's Office in the DHSS may be adequate for the Department's internal purposes but it has certainly not proved capable of supplying the informed customer for health research envisaged by Lord Rothschild.
>
> House of Lords, 1988, para.4.3

It therefore went on to recommend that an independent organisation – a National Health Research Authority – should be established to be

---

26. A more detailed account of policy development over the period than we can give here can be found in Culyer (1998).

responsible for most publicly funded research. The tasks proposed for it by the Committee are set out in the box below. The very length of the list reflects the scale of the Committee's dissatisfaction with the current situation.

PROPOSED FUNCTIONS OF THE NATIONAL HEALTH RESEARCH AUTHORITY

■ to identify on behalf of the NHS, and in consultation with medical research interests both public and private, those areas of research which should be given priority on the basis of service need

■ to ensure, in conjunction with the MRC, an adequate research capability for the needs of the NHS in clinical, public health and operational research

■ to commission research as necessary on behalf of the NHS

■ to advise on the implications of NHS policy and practice for medical research, including the training and career prospects of medical researchers, and where conflicts arise to ensure that the interests of research are fully taken into account

■ to provide a point of contact between the NHS and the MRC, the other Research Councils, the UGC, the Royal Colleges, the medical research charities, the pharmaceutical and medical equipment industries, and any others with medical research interests

■ to ensure that the results of research are efficiently disseminated and implemented within the NHS

■ to promote the evaluation of existing clinical practice and to under-take technology assessment of both new and current procedures

■ to promote systematic clinical audit (the evaluation of the appropriateness of treatment in specific cases)

■ to oversee the provision of statistical information for the NHS, in co-operation with the Office of Population Censuses and Surveys

■ to co-operate with the HEA in disseminating the results of research related to health promotion and the prevention of disease, with the Health and Safety Executive in occupational health and hygiene, and with the NHSTA in the training of NHS managers

■ to assist in co-ordinating the work of Regional Research Committees.

(House of Lords, 1988)

Directorate of R&D

The proposal for a freestanding authority was not accepted by the Conservative Government. Instead, an R&D programme was established within the Department of Health under a director of R&D who was 'expected to develop a research programme which meets the priority needs of the Department and the NHS'.

The terms of reference for the new directorate fell short of that proposed by the House of Lords Committee, but the new role was nevertheless a substantial one. In particular it promised to provide the central focus which the Nuffield analysis had identified as a serious gap.

In 1991 *Research for Health* was published, the first policy statement by the first Director of R&D, Michael Peckham (Department of Health, 1991a). This document is the second turning point in policy development. In very brief terms, it set out an entirely new prospectus for research funded by the Department of Health:

- *The R&D strategy for the NHS is part of a broader strategy for all aspects of R&D for which the Department of Health (DH) is responsible through the Director of Research and Development.*
- *The wider framework of the DH programme will be set in the context of the various determinants of health, and will ensure that R&D contributes fully to the objectives of Health of the Nation and the important task of setting clear, quantifiable health targets. The DH programme will include public health issues, including disease prevention, and the health sequelae of social and environmental factors and nutrition.*

    Department of Health, 1991a, p.2

If the Director of R&D was to fulfil his terms of reference, then he had to know 'what was going on' within his area of responsibility and have the means available for influencing the way in which the resources devoted to research were used. From the early 1990s onwards, a series of measures have aimed to put the Director and his successors in that position. The key has been reform of the way that financial resources are allocated to research. The rest of this chapter focuses on this process.

The central weakness, as far as the Director of R&D was concerned, was that in the early 1990s he could have no clear idea how much was being spent on R&D within the NHS and what it was being spent on. The 1988 report had clearly identified the confusion which prevailed over the current scale of spending. Although it had been possible to establish the broad pattern of spending in the health research economy as a whole, it proved more difficult to ascertain how much was then being spent within the NHS. There were various funding streams bearing on research, but no research budget as such and no comprehensive account of what was being spent by whom on what.

The 1988 report argued for what it termed 'hypothecation' of research funding, i.e. a ring-fenced allocation which would have provided an identifiable budget for health research within the ambit of the Department. But it did not spell out how exactly all the existing spending should be identified and then managed in line with centrally determined priorities.

The impact of the internal market and the Culyer report

This ring-fencing, as we shall see, required a substantial reform of NHS finances. However, the immediate impetus to financial reform came from elsewhere. In the early 1990s, fundamental changes were taking place in the organisation of the NHS. Implementation of the 1990 NHS and Community Care Act, which provided the foundation for an internal market in care services, began in 1991. This and other policies appeared to those in research-based trusts to be liable to make them uncompetitive in the market for health care, since they would be appear to be high-cost providers of care by virtue of their research activities.

The then President of the Royal Society wrote to the Prime Minister expressing his concern:

> I am writing to express the serious concern felt by my scientific colleagues about prospective developments in the Health Service and their potential impact on medical research and education. I hope that these concerns, which are very widely shared, will be addressed before it is too late.
>
> The long-standing excellence of medical education and research in the UK has been fostered by the close co-operation between Regional Health Authorities and their regional medical schools.
>
> If the Regional Health Authorities are reorganised or dissolved, then it is essential that the education and research which they currently

support should be financed through other channels. A further devolution of funds to individual purchasers, without adequate provision for the continued support of medical training and research, would lead to a serious crisis and a great loss of performance and reputation for British science.

House of Lords, 1995

The Government responded promptly to the concerns of the President.[27] A Task Force was set up under Professor Anthony Culyer to 'consider whether to recommend changes in the conduct and support of research and development in and by the NHS, and if so to advise on alternative funding and support mechanisms for R&D' (Department of Health, 1994).

TERMS OF REFERENCE FOR NHS R&D TASK FORCE

Taking into account the NHS Reforms and the functions and manpower review; and building on existing work, the Task Force is asked to:

i   take stock of the current situation with regard to the conduct and support of R&D in the NHS, to establish the nature and extent of any problems, and in that light to consider whether it is appropriate to make recommendations; and if it is

ii   review the ways in which the NHS currently funds its own R&D and supports that funded by others

iii   review the ways in which the NHS mechanisms for funding and supporting R&D promote and/or hinder the aims of the NHS R&D strategy and other Government policies relating to R&D in the NHS

iv   advise on alternative funding and support mechanisms for R&D, including any necessary transitional measures, recognising that any new system will have to operate within available resources.

(Department of Health, 1994, p.59)

---

27. The Government had already indicated that it would modify the formula for covering the 'excess' costs of teaching to include those of research, i.e. translating SIFT into SIFTR, a change which took place in 1990. However, the basis of the calculations remained obscure and it was not clear that the estimate of research costs was well founded. Although the 1988 House of Lords report attempted to estimate total spending on research, it found the situation within the NHS hard to fathom. A second House of Lords report noted the various attempts which had been made to estimate the R element of SIFTR and also the existence of what it called 'implicit research', following the term used in the Culyer report. But its scale eluded them.

In a subsequent paper, Culyer (1998) noted a series of problems with the financial arrangements in place when the Task Force began work:

- Some arrangements for the funding of research were temporary.
- SIFTR was a general hospital subsidy, more related to undergraduate numbers than R&D activity. It was not quality assessed and appeared to be poorly targeted on R&D activity within teaching hospitals, and was not available to support non-teaching institutions or community-based care.
- The pressures of the internal market threatened the funding of research currently met through contracts for patient services.
- There was evidence of a lack of co-operation in R&D projects from some fund-holding GPs.
- Referrals were increasingly local and increasingly difficult to obtain for major research centres.
- Service support for non-MRC research was not always available.
- There was inadequate co-ordination at the top level between different funders of R&D and an inadequate mechanism for identifying and prioritising the service needs of R&D.
- Much R&D in trusts was not evaluated or supported by explicit mechanisms.
- The reform of the NHS Executive was seen as a threat to the valuable work of the regional directors of R&D.

As this list indicates, the foundations for the development of a coherent NHS research strategy were far from being in place when the Task Force was established. The existing financial arrangements were not designed to support the role of the Director of R&D; there was no system for prioritising research areas; some of the infrastructure required for developing research projects (particularly clinical trials) was not in place; and there were no guarantees as to the quality of the work that was being done – indeed most was not monitored at all. Not surprisingly, therefore, the Task Force decided that radical measures were required.

Its report was based on three main points:

- *First, it is essential to separate funds for R&D and for service support for R&D from funds for other activity. Only by such a separation can health R&D be properly identified, managed and accounted for, and only by such greater clarity can one be sure that the investment in R&D will not be squeezed out as providers seek to keep their service prices to purchasers as low as possible.*

- *Second, those who perform R&D should justify their claims on resources, do so in competition with others, and be accountable for the R&D they do.*
- *Third, the primary and community care sectors should be put on an equal footing with the acute sector in terms of access to funding both for R&D and its associated service costs.*

Culyer, 1994a, p.1

As the third of these points indicates, it was recognised that the balance of research activity had to be changed, away from the traditional sites (the teaching and research hospitals) to community settings. In the early 1990s, the realisation was growing that much of the workload of the hospital could be carried out outside its walls – within general practice and the services associated with it. At a minimum, the new financial regime had to be capable of financing research supporting such a shift.

The Task Force's main financial proposal was that a levy system should be imposed on all purchasers, which would bring together all research funding within the NHS into a single stream:

> *11. We see no merit in maintaining all these disparate funding streams. We recommend that, with effect from 1995–96, a single explicit funding stream should replace the current diverse funding mechanisms, including the R of SIFTR, the research element of funding for the London Postgraduate hospitals, the Non-SIFTR scheme, other central and regional R&D and service support funds and, over time, most of health care providers' own account R&D.*

The change proposed is summed up in the box opposite.

As the box reveals, the new financial arrangements were intended both to clarify and simplify the existing muddle, allowing the identification of both the total budget and the broad purposes for which it was being used. The main new instrument was to be a levy on all health purchasers:

> *12. R&D is for the common good of the NHS, contributing in the long and short term to better quality and effectiveness in the health care provided on behalf of the resident population generally. Hence we recommend that this funding stream should be conceived as a levy on all health care purchasers' allocations and determined annually.*

FINANCIAL CHANGES PROPOSED BY THE TASK FORCE

Pre-Culyer	Post-Culyer (from 1996)
■ Central Research and Development Committee programme	■ Projects and programmes
■ Department of Health centrally-commissioned programme	■ Service support
■ Other Department of Health research	■ Research facilities
■ 25 per cent of SIFTR	■ Information systems
■ Non-SIFTR	■ Research capacity
■ Special health authorities' subvention	
■ Regional health authorities' R&D budgets	
■ 'Implicit research' (local purchasers and providers)	

This recommendation was accepted. Its implementation, however, has been protracted because the underpinnings required to introduce a levy were not in place in the early 1990s and in some respects not even by the end of the decade.

While the general pattern of research spending was known, i.e. its concentration in a small number of hospitals, particularly in London, no precise data were available on what each trust spent, nor on what research they funded. In 1995, therefore, the process of attempting to establish the current scale of research spending and activity within the NHS began. Trusts were required to declare the scale of their research activity as well as brief details of the projects they supported. According to a letter issued to chief executives of trusts in 1996 (Swales, 1996), some 39,000 projects had been identified, at a cost of £334 million.

Implementation of the Culyer proposals

A subsequent departmental paper (Department of Health, 1997d) set out the purpose of the levy – see the box overleaf. As the list indicates, the levy was intended not simply to fund research, but also to help provide the basis of a research capacity within the NHS – what it terms the infrastructure and environment. This was to provide the basis for both privately and publicly financed research, and also the capacity to use the results of that research. As Figure 3 (p.18) indicates, this support role is in fact more significant in expenditure terms than NHS research 'on own account'.

PURPOSE OF THE NHS R&D LEVY

- To meet the costs of the NHS's contribution to the infrastructure and environment in which health and health services R&D can flourish and be well managed. This includes contributing to the training of people intending to pursue R&D as an integral part of their career.
- To contribute to the development of the capacity of the NHS, and others, to identify needs for health and health services R&D, and to evaluate the costs and benefits of R&D.
- To meet certain costs incurred by providers of NHS services in supporting non-commercial R&D activity paid for by funders external to the NHS (e.g. charities, research councils).
- To allow providers of NHS services themselves to support, carry out or commission R&D of direct interest to the NHS.
- To commission, on behalf of the NHS as a whole, specific R&D activities identified as national or regional priorities for the service.
- To contribute to the dissemination of the findings of R&D.
- To make a contribution to encouraging the use and exploitation of R&D findings and the promotion of an evaluative and evidence-based culture in the policy and practice of the NHS, through the development and evaluation of techniques for implementing the results of R&D.

(Department of Health, 1997d)

In early 1997 the Department of Health issued *R&D Support Funding for NHS Providers*, the next step towards the creation of a new financial system. This indicated that there would be two forms of funding financed from the levy:

- R&D support funding for providers, i.e. NHS trusts or other health services bodies
- the centrally managed NHS R&D programme

The first of these was itself divided into two:

> **Portfolio Funding** *is intended for those Providers who are able to predict their funding needs over several years, and take a strategic approach to managing their R&D activity. It will be a block of funds to meet all the Provider's R&D Support costs. Providers will have considerable discretion to use the funds as they think best. It will be awarded for four years at a time (three years for the first round of funding starting in April 1998).*
>
> **Task-Linked Funding** *will be for any period up to four years. Providers will receive a single block of funding, but unlike Portfolio Funding this will usually be broken down into two or more 'Tasks' or areas of activity. These 'Tasks' can range from one or two projects in a small Provider, through to the R&D activity of one or more hospital specialties or departments.*
>
> Department of Health, 1997e, p.5

Portfolio funding for providers 'able to predict their funding needs over several years' clearly fitted the needs of existing research trusts with established research programmes, while task-linked funding for specific task or projects allowed newcomers to enter into research at modest levels of commitment.

The second stream, the NHS R&D programme, was to be used to fund centrally commissioned programmes of work and eight regional programmes. Work commissioned centrally on behalf of the NHS was to reflect national priorities, while regional programmes were to be used for both regional and nationally identified needs. As the table overleaf shows, however, expenditure on these was modest. The bulk of the budget therefore remained within the NHS.

Because of the risk of upsetting the finance of trusts with substantial research programmes, the Culyer report suggested that 'For 1995–96 there should be no significant departure from the existing sums or the present principles for distribution.' (Culyer, 1994a). From 1997/98 onwards, a process of gradual reallocation began, first to bring levy monies into line with the amounts of research declared – some trusts declaring research programmes received nothing under the earlier arrangements – and second, from 1998/99 onwards, to begin to shift levy proceeds away from the existing research-intensive trusts towards other hospital and community-based institutions.

TABLE 5: NATIONAL PROGRAMME EXPENDITURE 1995/96

PROGRAMME	£
Mental health	1,415,151
Cardiovascular disease and stroke	3,093,223
Physical and complex disabilities	1,512,600
Primary/secondary care interface	1,934,000
Cancer	298,500
Mother and child health	40,000
Implementation methods	40,000
Health technology assessment	2,026,747
Total	**10,360,221**

Before the process of implementation was far advanced, the House of Lords Select Committee took another look at research funding in *Medical Research and the NHS Reforms* (House of Lords, 1995). In contrast to its earlier report, it was upbeat, commending most of the changes which had been made. The Culyer proposals were broadly welcomed, as was the R&D strategy itself. Its main conclusion was that:

> *A great deal has been achieved ... towards meeting the need which this Committee identified in 1988 for the NHS to engage actively with the research community. ... Of all the NHS reforms since 1990, the R&D strategy is certainly the one least widely known; but, among those who are aware of it, it is, we suspect, the one most unequivocally welcomed.*

House of Lords, 1995, para.2.2

In its response to the report the Government welcomed:

> *the constructive spirit in which the Committee, through the Report, offers its detailed recommendations and conclusions. The Report – and this Response – shows that concerns about R&D and the new patient care arrangements in the NHS have been heeded, and are being addressed.*

Department of Health, 1995g, p.1

This 'exchange' would seem to indicate that all was progressing well. Nevertheless, it soon became apparent that the new arrangements were still not adequate. In 1997 the Central Research and Development Committee (CRDC) commissioned a strategic review of the levy. The resulting report (Department of Health, 1999a) concluded that although a lot had been achieved following its introduction, further changes were needed. Its central conclusions did not bear directly on finance, but it is apparent from their nature that the process of reform was still far from complete.

The review report is very brief, but it contains a number of substantial criticisms of the way that the management of the R&D budget was developing. In particular it found that:

- a clearer focus on NHS needs and priorities was needed
- improved quality assurance systems for research programmes were required
- there should be systematic involvement of wider health communities and consumers in NHS R&D
- research capacity in terms of research training and career prospects needed to be developed.

We will pick up on all these themes in this and the following two chapters. Suffice to say now that it sparked off a great deal of activity designed to deal with the major weaknesses it identified.

Proposals for two funding streams

As far as finance is concerned, the Department of Health responded with a series of papers published in 2000, a policy paper, *Research and Development for a First Class Service: R&D funding in the new NHS*, and two consultation papers (Department of Health, 2000e and 2000g) which foreshadowed further reforms both of how priorities within publicly financed research are determined and of how such research is financed.

As far as funding is concerned, the papers proposed the division of funding for NHS research within the 'service support' element of the budget into two streams: NHS Priorities and Needs Funding, and Support for Science.

NHS Priorities and Needs Funding is intended to support:

- the implementation of the NHS priorities in National Priorities Guidance

- the programme of national service frameworks and the National Performance Assessment Framework
- the work of the National Institute for Clinical Excellence
- the needs of the NHS in implementing Government policy.

It is also designed to 'build up and support':

- public health R&D and epidemiology
- R&D in primary care
- clinical research on new treatments, and other work to develop and apply new technology for the public good where there is no commercial sponsor
- health services research on innovation, treatment and organisational issues in all health care setting.

NHS Support for Science is designed to meet the NHS costs of supporting R&D under agreed standards of strategic direction and quality assurance by the research councils and other eligible R&D funding partners. It therefore includes, where appropriate, an element for the costs of developing R&D proposals and for building work around that supported by the external funder.

The relationship between the new and the old arrangements is shown in Figure 6, opposite.

As with the Culyer levy, the new financial system could not be implemented immediately. Instead, the existing levy system was effectively put on hold, i.e. budgets were rolled forward, until the new arrangements could be brought in.

Inadequacies in information

In any case, one crucial element remained to be determined before introduction of the division between the two main funding streams: how much of the budget should go into each. The basis for the decision was unavailable: existing financial information did not make the required distinction. It was not even clear that funds nominally dedicated to research were in fact being spent on research. A report by the Science and Technology Committee of the House of Commons, *Cancer Research: A fresh look* (House of Commons, 2000) notes 'the conviction of many witnesses ... that most of the R&D funding was disappearing into general support for NHS hospitals and that little of it was actually made available

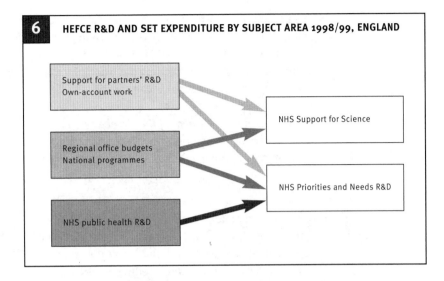

6   HEFCE R&D AND SET EXPENDITURE BY SUBJECT AREA 1998/99, ENGLAND

for research purposes'. It found this situation 'deeply unsatisfactory'. The Government's response (Department of Health, 2000c) fell short of offering reassurance that the evidence received by the Committee was wrong.

Similarly a research report on the implementation of the Culyer reforms found that:

> *existing cost measurement and accounting systems have proved inadequate for the purpose of tracking and managing R&D support costs at the operational level.*

> Arnold *et al.*, 1999, p.1

In recognition of deficiencies such as these the Department of Health commissioned the study from MHA consultants to help in the design of the new system. The consultants were charged with developing an Activity and Cost model which would examine the activities currently being undertaken in support of externally funded R&D and their associated costs and use these to provide the basis for developing the funding system. In their interim report the consultants commented:

> *The invitation to tender and the original project plan assumed that there would be sufficient data available in providers to be able to undertake a robust data collection and analysis exercise.*

> MHA, 2000, p.10

This assumption proved misplaced. Further work was required before a protocol could be issued to the NHS indicating how this funding element was to be calculated (reported in MHA, 2002). In 2001, the Department of Health issued a statement setting out what information those receiving funding would have to supply. As it says:

> The sound management of R&D in health and social care depends on accurate and comprehensive information about research activity and, therefore, on good information management systems.

Department of Health, 2001n, p.1

Once again, therefore, the financial system was largely 'frozen'. Given that the new system itself will take time to bed down, it will be some time before substantial changes in the use of the levy funds in their new form can be made – indeed a paper setting out the transitional arrangement for 2001/02 (Department of Health, 2001l) indicated that it would not be until 2003/04 that allocations would be changed in the light of strategic reviews covering (not for the first time) cancer, coronary disease and mental health – the so-called priority areas in the NHS Plan.[28] The paper acknowledges (para.5.1) that: 'It will take some time for the mature systems for NHS Priorities and Needs R&D funding to evolve.' The same is true of Support for Science. It follows that the financial system for support of research within the NHS remains in a state of transition as it has been in since the mid-1990s.

The total budget

The 1988 report concluded that too little was being spent on medical research:

> 2.72 Several witnesses made the point that was put succinctly by Sir Walter Bodmer: 'It is little less than appalling that a department with an approximately £20 thousand million annual expenditure on the Health Service funds a research programme of its own at a level hardly more than £20 million. Indeed, the overall expenditure on medical research (outside the pharmaceutical industry) is of the order of £300 million, namely only about 1.5 per cent of the Health Service Budget, a level which would be considered totally inadequate by

---

28. The timetable set out in this paper superseded that set out in *Research and development for a first class service*.

most major pharmaceutical companies to guarantee their medium to long term future. This emphasises the need not only to increase considerably the direct resources within the Department of Health for research relevant to the application of advances to new approaches to prevention, diagnosis and treatment, but also to increase the overall research expenditure base which, as always emphasised, provides so many new and exciting possibilities for significant practical advances.'

House of Lords, 1988, p.314

Research for Health (Department of Health, 1991a) proposed that Department of Health/NHS spending on research should rise from its current level (estimated to be just under 1 per cent of the NHS budget) to 1.5 per cent over a period of five years. Sir Michael Peckham subsequently indicated to the House of Lords Committee that this should not be regarded as a rigid target. As we have seen, at the time it was set there was very little knowledge available about how much was being spent on what. Although the 1988 Committee was able to establish the broad outline of the health research economy as it then stood, it was not able to penetrate far into the NHS itself. Unsurprisingly, there was very limited work focused on trying to determine how productive the research was.

A number of projects designed to measure the value of research were funded during the 1990s, including a series of pilots carried out by the Health Economics Research Unit at Brunel University. But, as Buxton and Hanney (1994) have shown in their review of this and other work, the obstacles to achieving effective evaluation are severe. They concluded that:

> *It is certainly too early to answer the question as to whether the NHS R&D programme will give value for money, but it is possible to draw some conclusions, partly from analysis of research funded before the start of the NHS R&D programme. It has been possible to estimate the nature, and to a degree the extent, of payback from some past projects or programmes, particularly those aimed at particular policy issues. However, it has also been possible to identify projects that had virtually no payback. It is clear that good science is necessary but is not sufficient.*

Against this background, it is not surprising that very little has been published by those responsible for NHS and other centrally funded R&D as to the benefits of the programme as a whole, i.e. the kind of evidence on which one might base a judgement as to the appropriate scale of the programme. Nor is there, in the public domain at least, any indication of the technical merits of proposals which are not receiving funding.

In 2001 the Wellcome Trust, in conjunction with the London Regional Office, published *Putting NHS Research on the Map* (NHS Executive, 2001). This did not aim to demonstrate 'value for money', but, using the bibliometric techniques the Trust had used for its own programme (Dawson *et al.*, 1998), it aimed to show what the NHS programmes were producing by way of published outputs and what their impact, as measured by citations, had been.

As the authors recognise, this work represents a beginning rather than a conclusion: in particular, the impact on clinical practice eluded them, although they make suggestions as to how this might be captured. They point out that nearly all the basic research carried out within the NHS is funded externally, but that the link between this and clinical advance is not clear. They therefore conclude that 'there is an urgent need to develop our understanding in this area' (NHS Executive, 2001, p.38).

Just so. The very fact that this study did not appear until 2001, and then with the support of a private foundation, indicates just how little attention has been given so far by the Department of Health to the value of the health research it finances within the NHS.

The absence of such evidence in itself does not demonstrate that the programme is too large, or not large enough. But it leaves the NHS programme open to the criticism that it is what it is because it has always been there. Nevertheless, in February 2001 it was announced that the NHS R&D budget would be increased by 6.6 per cent to £479 million, of which more than £400 million would go directly to the NHS (Department of Health, 2001d).

Given the scale of the total NHS budget and the rate of clinical change (driven partly by the private sector, but also influenced by the Government reforms), a budget of this size seems, intuitively, more likely to be too small than to be too large,[29] particularly since, as the figures in Chapter 1 indicate, such a small proportion of the total budget is geared directly to the NHS. Intuition is scarcely the proper basis for long-term policy making, but at the moment there is little else to go on.

---

29. See material at: www.laskerfoundation.org on the value of medical research.

Overview

As this very condensed account indicates, the process of financial reform begun in the early 1990s is far from complete. Indeed, although the introduction of the levy has succeeded in making the funding for NHS internal R&D explicit at national and local levels, little of substance has changed since the reforms began. Essentially the system remains in transition, though the end point of the transition is different from that envisaged when the reforms began.

We have shown that the system by which resources are allocated to R&D within the NHS rests on inadequate foundations. It remains unclear just what the resources nominally devoted to research actually purchase – indeed it still remains unclear whether they are *all* used for research.

The consultation documents issued in 2000 and 2001 acknowledge the deficiencies of the system, embodying as they do new proposals for the allocation of research finance at both the strategic level and the project or programme level. The new requirements to provide information imposed on those receiving funding should provide a better basis for decisions made under the new system.

The changes under way promise that in due course the Department of Health will be much better placed to determine how NHS research funding is used. As the current Director of R&D put it in a letter to chief executives issued in February 2001:

> *There will be some devils in the detail but I think [we will be able] to deliver funding systems that meet the needs of the NHS and its partners.*

Pattison, 2001

These are just now coming into place. Hence, after the best part of a decade of financial reform, the Department of Health still does not have the financial machinery it requires if is to influence, in the light of its priorities, the content of all the work it currently finances. The question which follows is: Is the Department in a position to use that ability once it is achieved? This is the subject of the next chapter.

Chapter 4

The balance of spending

One of the criticisms made by the House of Lords in 1988 was that research providers had too much influence on the pattern of publicly funded research. This chapter examines moves to include a wider range of voices in determining priorities. It finds, nevertheless, that broad areas continue to be neglected and that the Department of Health lacks a general set of principles to guide the allocation of research funds.

4 The balance of spending

This chapter focuses on the Department of Health R&D spending, including central, regional and NHS budgets. Following the objectives set for it in the first edition of *Research for Health*, we assume that the aim of the programme as a whole is to make the maximum possible contribution to the 'health of the nation' by improving the care offered through the NHS or by supporting attempts by the Department of Health or other parts of Government to reduce the incidence of ill health. The task of those controlling the R&D programme is to select, or support the means of selecting, the disposition of the funds which is most likely to achieve that 'maximum possible contribution'.

This task cannot be carried out in a mechanistic way, relying purely on accepted techniques for valuing specific research projects or bids for funds (Buxton and Hanney, 1994). Our emphasis in this chapter is not in any case on specific projects, but rather on the broad balance of spending on research, the means used to change that balance when required and, following the analysis of Chapter 2, any systematic or persistent gaps or biases in the way that the overall programme is made up. As in the previous chapter we begin with the House of Lords 1988 report and then consider the steps that have been taken to remedy what it saw as imbalances in the composition of spending at the end of the 1980s.

Early days

The 1988 report found that there were no arrangements for identifying gaps or setting research priorities across the health research economy as a whole:

> *remarkably there appears to be no coherent means of setting priorities beyond that which is provided by the MRC in discussions with the*

DHSS ... The only body which appears to accept some responsibility for supporting underfunded areas of research is the Wellcome Trust. The Committee do not believe that Governments should rely on charities to fill gaps in national research effort.

House of Lords, 1988, para.3.15

At the time the report was written, there was no systematically presented information on what the NHS was spending and still less on what it was doing with the funds at its disposal. Even though the Department of Health *Yearbook of Research and Development 1990* does contain an account of the contents of the programme at that time (see box below), the areas of research listed do not amount to a systematically defined set of programmes supporting all the Department of Health's activities. Rather, they reflect a mix of service and management concerns and do not cover what was being funded within the NHS by any of the more or less explicit routes referred to in Chapter 3.

The House of Lords Committee clearly recognised that the research funded by the then Department of Health and Social Security for its own purposes or for the NHS should be seen as part of a wider research economy and its role and composition determined in the light of that

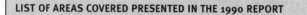

LIST OF AREAS COVERED PRESENTED IN THE 1990 REPORT

- AIDS
- Child Care
- Research Units:
  Blind Mobility Research Unit
  Centre for Primary Care Research
  National Perinatal Epidemiology Unit
  Social Medicine and Health Services Research Unit
  Social Policy Research Unit
  Unit of Clinical Epidemiology
- Health and Personal Social Services Research Programme
- Information Technology
- Procurement

(Department of Health, 1990)

broader context. But, as the Committee found, there was at that time no organisation, not even the Department itself, which tried to take such a view. The Wellcome Trust was playing what we defined in Chapter 2 as one of the State's central roles, as were other charities in a smaller way. But these could not take on all the roles we defined, particularly the needs of the NHS as a deliverer of care.

The Committee received evidence from a wide range of witnesses which enabled it to identify a number of broad areas – molecular biology, clinical research, public health and operational research – and disciplines where little research was being conducted. Nearly all the research then being funded was in support of medicine to the detriment of the other professions whose members were, of course, vastly more numerous.

Within medicine itself, the need was to ensure that at least part of the resources being devoted to research took into account the needs of the NHS as a deliverer of care:

> The NHS should be brought into the mainstream of medical research. It should articulate its research needs; it should assist in meeting those needs; and it should ensure that the fruits of research are systematically transferred into service.
>
> House of Lords, 1988, para.4.4–7

The last of these is not just a matter of dissemination but rather of linking the 'lab to the patient', i.e. clinical, patient-focused research, the second of the general 'gaps' listed above.[30]

As for more narrowly defined areas, the report set out a long list of topics which individuals or organisations giving evidence perceived as being neglected. It did not endorse these very numerous specific claims, but at a minimum they represented a widespread dissatisfaction with the balance of areas being funded. Some voices, it would seem, were not being heard when funds were being allocated to research even where, as the list indicates, there was already an established research tradition, such as in the field of cancer.

---

30. It would probably not conclude now that molecular biology was a neglected area.

NEGLECTED AREAS IDENTIFIED IN THE 1988 REPORT

- Ageing
- Alzheimer's disease
- Anaesthesia
- Asthma
- Back pain
- Blindness
- Bronchitis, emphysema and other lung diseases
- Cancer
- Cardiovascular disease
- Children's diseases
- Clinical pharmacokinetics
- Cochlear implants
- Complementary medicine
- Congenital mental disorders
- Deafness
- Dental caries and periodontal disease
- Diabetes
- Epidemiology
- Gland disorders
- Health promotion and preventive medicine
- Mental handicap
- Midwifery
- Mucosal disease
- Neonatal disorders and perinatal morbidity
- Nursing
- Nutrition
- Optometry
- Oral cancer
- Osteoporosis
- Parkinson's disease
- Pathology
- Pharmacy
- Psychiatry
- Rheumatism
- Schizophrenia
- Sexually-transmitted diseases
- Skin cancer, skin diseases
- Spastics
- Stroke
- Tropical medicine
- Kidney disease

(House of Lords, 1988)

Policy response

The appointment of a director of R&D within the Department of Health was the first institutional response to the 1988 report's analysis. This appointment was followed by the establishment of the CRDC to support the new director: its terms of reference are set out in the box opposite.

As far as we have been able to establish, neither the CRDC nor the R&D directorate attempted at the time of their formation to take a view on the overall disposition of research resources and how it might be changed in the light of its view of what the NHS required and in the light of what other parts of the health research economy were doing. Instead, the

---

CRDC INITIAL TERMS OF REFERENCE

To advise the Director of Research and Development, and through him the NHS Management Executive, on priorities within a national strategic framework for a multidisciplinary R&D programme to improve the scientific basis of the use of health care resources.

1. areas in which R&D would be of value to the NHS, distinguishing between:
    a   a number of areas of national priority which merit central NHS funding
    b   other areas of national importance on which NHS R&D should focus
    c   NHS needs that might be drawn to the attention of other funders, such as the MRC
2. goals and objectives for work funded by the NHS in priority areas
3. evaluation of the outcomes of research programmes against these goals
4. methods of improving the utility and utilisation of research results
5. the infrastructure for research, including:
    a   services support for research
    b   R&D information systems for the NHS to co-ordinate research planning and ensure effective dissemination of results
6. any other matters relating to research and development on which the DRD may ask for guidance.

(DOH, 1995f)

CRDC set up a series of time-limited research committees charged with determining research priorities in the following areas:

- mental health and learning disabilities
- cardiovascular disease and stroke
- physical and complex disabilities
- primary and secondary care interface
- cancer
- mother and child health
- primary dental care
- asthma management
- methods of implementing research findings.

Each of these reviews produced reports over the next two to three years which identified priorities in their fields. Programmes of research duly followed, financed from the centrally financed element of the NHS R&D programme. These programmes, as the figures set out in Chapter 3 indicated, were modest in scope. More significantly, the exercise as a whole did not bite on the bulk of the funds then being used for research within the NHS either in these specific fields or overall.

Furthermore although some of the areas remained 'priorities' and were reviewed again, others did not. For example, a programme of work on the primary/secondary interface was commissioned and the results reported (Department of Health, 1999g). But this was the end, rather than the beginning of an attempt to understand how the various parts of the NHS meshed or did not mesh with each other and what the benefits of change in their respect roles might be. This was despite the fact that the issues remained as important a decade later as they had been when the area was initially identified.[31]

Although the subject area reviews were wound up, as noted above, another, smaller series was commissioned in the second half of the 1990s following work carried out under the auspices of CRDC to determine 'strategic priorities'. These covered cancer (again), accidents,

---

THE MAIN CENTRAL PROGRAMMES

In 1996 the centrally run programmes were rationalised into three elements: the Health Technology Assessment Programme (HTA), the Service Delivery and Organisation Programme (SDO) and the New and Emerging Technologies Programme (NEAT), while the Policy Research Programme (the old Centrally Commissioned Programme relabelled) continued in place.

HTA's main role is to respond, using the available research, to specific questions to which clinicians require answers when delivering care – a response to one of the criticisms from the 1988 report bearing on the links between research and practice.

continued opposite

---

31. In fact these programmes are still (partly) alive, as a visit to the R&D website will show.

THE MAIN CENTRAL PROGRAMMES *continued*

HTA is the successor of the health technology standing group established in 1991. Although often described in R&D papers as 'the centrepiece of the NHS R&D programme', its focus is on the evaluation of health technologies:

> *to ensure that high quality research information on the costs, effectiveness and broader impact of health technologies is produced in the most efficient way for those who use, manage and work in the NHS.*

The programme is described as being needs-led, i.e. it aims at responding to those who have to use its results (NHS Executive, 1999, p.1).

NEAT (originally NET) is intended to 'promote the use of new and emerging technologies to develop new medical products and clinical interventions to enhance the efficiency and effectiveness of health and social care' (Department of Health, 1995f, p.17.1). This is a small programme funding only a handful of projects.

SDO appeared in official papers as long ago as 1996, but it was only launched formally in 2000. Its terms of reference are to:

- ensure that good research-based evidence about the responsiveness, effectiveness, cost-effectiveness and equity of different models of service is available and accessible
- generate the evidence base to encourage health service managers and others to implement appropriate change
- identify and develop appropriate R&D methods
- promote the development of expert R&D capacity
- involve service users and other stakeholders in the programme.
(Dalziel, 2000, p.5)

In addition the Policy Research Programme aims:

> *to provide, through high quality research, a knowledge base for health services policy, social services policy and central policies directed at the health of the population as a whole.*

> Department of Health, 1997c, p.3

ageing, cardio-vascular disease and stroke, and primary care. The subjects were chosen to support what were then seen as national priorities in the light of the aims set out in *The Health of the Nation* (Department of Health, 1991b).

In 1997, the CRDC commissioned a review of the levy system. The review concluded that 'the needs of the NHS' were still attracting too little attention. It therefore made three general and fundamental recommendations:

- *the Central Research & Development Committee should establish time limited national research advisory groups in research priority areas to foster relevant comprehensive research across all constituent health communities*
- *the Department of Health as a strategic funder of research and development should maintain a rolling programme of reviews to establish strategic priorities for research*
- *the Department of Health should promote ways of developing cross departmental research programme where these benefit the public health.*

Department of Health, 1999a

These recommendations might be taken as indicating that the process of finding the 'best possible mix' of projects had scarcely begun, even in those areas considered to be national priorities. They suggest that the review committee considered that the subject area reviews had not succeeded in identifying which subjects were most important, that a proper process had yet to be established across the health field as a whole and that links with other departments had been neglected. That harsh indictment was confirmed in the reports of the five reviews referred to above, which also found that even in the very fundamental areas covered, a systematic approach was yet to be found.

To give examples: the review of ageing found the field in disarray; while endorsing the MRC review of ageing (MRC, 1994b), it was 'disappointed to conclude that despite efforts by the MRC, little improvement has emerged in the national research portfolio' (Department of Health, 1999c, para.5.1.1). The review of cardiovascular disease and stroke found that, despite decades of research, new areas of work should be addressed and it went on to conclude that:

*The current R&D programme does not currently provide a
management structure to get the best return from England's
national research resource.*

Department of Health, 1999e, p.12

The review of accidents (Department of Health, 1999h) raised a different
issue. While emphasising the need for collaborative research, it
concluded that 'Responsive programmes … do not tend to attract the kind
of research necessary to develop sustainable collaborations'. In other
words, despite identification of accidents as a priority area, an
appropriate commissioning structure for research in it had not been
established when this review was completed.

Furthermore, according to the second topic review of primary care, the
project basis of most funding hindered the accumulation of 'knowledge in
a continuous way, testing the conclusions of research and building new
studies on the basis of previous ones' (Department of Health, 1999g,
section 3.2.2).

In other words, there was no mechanism or institution in a position to
take a continuing and effective overview of the whole field. The review of
cardiovascular disease and stroke (Department of Health, 1999e) made a
similar point. Its report strongly supports other groups in proposing a
national strategic R&D framework designed to co-ordinate and support
the whole research and practitioner community, rather than simply giving
grants for specific research topics.[32]

In brief, these reports suggest that a systematic and strategic approached
had yet to be developed in any of these areas despite their political and
scientific prominence. Against that background, there can be no reason to
believe that at the time they were being prepared the Department was
able, against any set of criteria, to argue that the projects it was then
supporting represented the 'best possible' deployment of the funds at
its disposal.

---

32. We make no comments here on the cancer topic report since we refer to this in Chapter 7:
suffice to say here that, despite its prominence, this area of research was also found to be
poorly co-ordinated.

The recent response

As with finance, the criticisms made by the strategic review of the levy received a substantial response. In 2000 the Department of Health paper *Research and Development for a First Class Service* set out 'the steps that the Department will take to obtain expert advice to inform work to clarify the strategic direction of research in and for the NHS'. This involved establishing:

> expert advisory structures to advise on R&D priorities and needs in particular topics and how these can best be addressed. These structures will address needs for R&D collaborations, capacity and infrastructure as well as specific projects and programmes of work. They will advise on needs in both the short and longer term.

> Department of Health, 2000b, p.19

Subsequently groups were established on cancer, on heart disease and stroke and on mental health, the three priority areas identified in the NHS Plan and other official documents and within which specific targets for health improvement had been set.

The subsequent consultation paper *NHS R&D Funding: NHS priorities and needs R&D funding* (Department of Health, 2000e) set out the Government's view on how priorities should be determined and the need for research identified. The arrangements embody two main elements:

- strategic priorities, which stem from current Government policies, e.g. national service frameworks
- broader NHS needs.

As far as the first of these is concerned, it reaffirms that cancer, coronary heart disease and mental health will continue to be the main priority areas. As for the second, the paper describes how the NHS and others will be involved in determining 'the needs of the NHS' and sets out the range of work to be included:

> 3.10 The scope of work required to develop the knowledge base for the NHS ... includes:

> - secondary research to synthesise existing research findings about a particular treatment, service, management question or other health issue

■ *primary research to strengthen knowledge*
■ *development of innovative treatments and technologies, and translation of them into practice.*

Department of Health, 2000e, p.6

The list itself is so general that it has little substantive content and no one could disagree with it. But it provides no indication of whether the current balance between these activities is deemed to be incorrect, nor does it make any attempt to define specific topics within these broad areas. In other words, this paper, like others appearing during 2000 and 2001, are largely concerned with process, at a very general level, rather the 'real' task of identifying what research should be done.

In 2001, a companion paper identifying the research needs of the public health function was published (Department of Health, 2001c). The paper is also very non-specific both about where more research would be worthwhile and about the means of determining how such areas could be identified:

5.8 Identifying threats to public health and opportunities for health improvement usually engenders a large requirement for new research. Funders will use criteria for prioritising topics which include likely impact on health and well being, urgency and timeliness, feasibility, and usefulness for implementation. At the same time strategic issues must be considered and a broad picture of public health and the ability of R&D to improve it maintained and developed.

Department of Health, 2001c, p.20

Although the very publication of this paper represents an advance over the situation revealed in the 1988 report, its actual content, as this extract suggests, is essentially rhetorical, not substantive.

The lack of substantive content in all the papers issued in the last two years can be attributed to the Department of Health's focus on improving the machinery for programme management in the light of the findings of the review of the levy system. But the very nature of these papers means that the criticisms from the 1988 report bearing on the content of the R&D programme remain to be addressed. Improvement in process – at least as far as the mechanisms for allocating funds is concerned – appears to be under way: what about substance?

Gaps in research

At the start of this chapter we noted the long list of specific 'gaps' recorded in the 1988 report and the shorter list of general gaps the House of Lords Committee itself endorsed. The situation identified in 1988 appeared to the Committee to be one of such gross imbalance that the need for some degree of reallocation of resources seemed self-evident. The long list of gaps recorded in the box on p.84 represents a list of 'claims' by individuals or organisations for their own areas of work or interest. It would be inappropriate simply to assume either that these gaps 'should' be filled, or that the list was comprehensive.

But even if we accepted the list of topics as *prima facie* candidates for being 'under-researched', it is impossible, from existing sources, to identify easily or comprehensively how much, in terms of spending or any other measure, is being devoted to these fields now. The Department of Health R&D website contains the National Research Projects Register, which contains details of thousands of completed projects or projects which are under way. However, much of the required information, e.g. on spending or source of funding, is missing.

Furthermore the Department of Health has not issued any analysis of its own of the current disposition of research resources even within its own ambit – because it has yet to obtain the information required to do so across all areas of spending. It is impractical therefore to revisit the 1988 list and see what has happened within each area on it.

Instead we will take a small number of topics which on the basis of recent reviews or other sources, might be regarded as 'under-researched'. The aim is not to be exhaustive, but rather to illustrate the progress, or lack of it, that has been made towards the goal implicitly set in 1988 of relating the research funded by the Department of Health and the NHS to the needs of the NHS.

There is no unique set of criteria which can be used to determine whether an area is or is not under-researched. Whether cancer attracts too much funding relative to Parkinson's cannot be determined purely by reference to the facts about the scale and nature of these conditions and the results of recent research. It is not our purpose to make particular cases of this kind.

However, it is reasonable to turn to the general principles which underpin the NHS and consider whether research has been commissioned to support their realisation. Of these, the most important is equal access for equal need. This can be expressed another way: when decisions are made as to whom to treat, a range of criteria are not relevant (the most obvious being age, sex and ethnicity) while others (such as clinical need or urgency) are relevant. Of these we take age.

The needs of older people

In 2001 the Government issued instructions to the NHS to carry out an audit to determine whether or not it was discriminating against elderly people in the delivery of care. Such discrimination as exists is sometimes the result of explicit policy, e.g. age cut-offs for access to certain treatments. However, it may also be implicit, arising from day-to-day decisions on individual cases. A King's Fund study found that there was widespread perception that age discrimination remains endemic in the NHS (Roberts *et al.*, 2002).

The study did not extend to research, but essentially the same scope for bias exists here. A review of access to cardiac rehabilitation services found strong *prima facie* evidence for discrimination in provision of services, but it also found that the underlying research base was very limited (Whelan, 1998). This in turn meant that it could not be shown, using the available evidence, that older people could benefit from the range of services reviewed in the report (see, for example, Grimley Evans, 1997).

The review of ageing cited above suggests that this is in part due to a systematic bias in the way that research is carried out:

> *We have noted ... that older people are still being excluded from trials of drugs and other interventions from which they might benefit. One reason is a fear that their 'frailty' will lead to unacceptable incidence or severity of side-effects. This should not be assumed without good evidence as there are abundant reports of good results from even major interventions for older people.*

Department of Health, 1999c, p.20

Elderly people use health services more intensively than younger people and account for about half of hospital bed-days. They are also heavy users of the primary care pharmaceuticals budget. If research programmes started from care needs, it is hard to see how biases of the kind identified above could arise.[33, 34]

This point has been recognised in recent guidance. The R&D Research Governance Framework states that:

> *2.2.7 Research and those pursuing it should respect the diversity of human culture and conditions and take full account of ethnicity, gender, disability, age and sexual orientation in its design, undertaking, and reporting. Researchers should take account of the multi-cultural nature of society. It is particularly important that the body of research evidence available to policy makers reflects the diversity of the population*

Department of Health, 2001e, p.11

Furthermore, the MRC guidelines on trial design now state:

> *Age and Gender: We require that, in full proposals, any proposed lower and upper age limits for trial participants should be justified on scientific grounds. Normally, for example, there should be no upper age limit on recruitment. Similarly, exclusion on the grounds of gender should be justifiable on scientific grounds*

MRC, 2001, p.4

The first of the above quotes is extremely vague: it scarcely amounts to a declaration of intent to ensure that the research done actually applies to all sections of the population, including older people. The second is more precise, but there are indications that in practice trials are not carried out in a way which removes discrimination (King's Fund, 2000b). The point applies to children as well as to elderly people (see European Health Management Association, 2001).

---

33. The needs of older people have of course been recognised in numerous pieces of individual research and the MRC has published an overview (see MRC, 1994 and also DTI/OST, 1995).

34. See, for example, Wenger (1992) who makes the point vividly: 'When the police queried the notorious criminal Willie Sutton as to why he robbed banks he replied, "because that's where the money is". Similarly data applicable to elderly patients and to women must be derived from the relevant research source: studies conducted in these specific populations.' In other words, if you are seeking to create health gain, this is where to look.

However, the main issue is not trial design, though that is important, but rather that, as things stand, the composition of current programmes embodies an implicit and largely unexamined assumption that older people are unlikely to be able to benefit as much as younger people.

Not surprisingly, therefore, the ageing topic review found little evidence of direction in the field as a whole. It concluded that 'a directed NHS strategy for research relevant to the health and social needs of the ageing population was necessary.' (Department of Health, 1999c). That conclusion is in itself obvious enough, given the well-known demographic changes in the UK population. The only surprise perhaps is that it took until 1999 for the NHS R&D programme to produce a (published) report which embodied it.[35]

The research community as a whole was well aware that research was necessary to anticipate and prepare for the consequences of demographic change. But the topic review found that:

> for too many topics there is little sense of purpose of direction in the body of research as a whole. Studies are repetitious and with the exception of occasional corpora from individual investigators or groups, studies do not build on what has gone before.

Department of Health, 1999c, p.12

In other words, the field lacked the strategic direction that a well-organised R&D programme might have been expected to give it.

Since the review was completed, the national service framework for older people has been published (Department of Health, 2001g). This states that:

> The overarching aims of the R&D strategy for older people will be to support research on how to:
>
> ■ reduce disability and the need for long-term care by maximising independent living and social functioning and improving rehabilitation services

---

35. *Growing older* (Department of Health and Social Security, 1981) claimed to be the first comprehensive review of all the issues bearing on the well-being of elderly people. It contains a paragraph on research which briefly refers to the then existing machinery for encouraging it. However, it contains no proposals for areas requiring research – proposals which might have been expected to emerge from such a comprehensive review.

- *enhance the well-being of older people and their carers and promote understanding of the needs of older people from black and minority ethnic communities*
- *inform the choices of individual users of health and social care services*
- *provide those who deploy health and social care resources with knowledge about the most cost-effective and equitable means of meeting those choices and best practice*
- *encourage the development and evaluation of innovative practice in health and social care.*

Department of Health, 2001g, para.33

The paper adds that:

Research on older people will respect the diversity of human culture and conditions and take full account of ethnicity, gender, disability, age and sexual orientation in its design, undertaking and reporting.

By implication it accepts that this has not been done in the past. Furthermore, the proposal for new machinery (see the box opposite) implies the absence of an effective means of defining and commissioning work in this field. In other words, reiteration of the need for research in this area and new arrangements for commissioning only serve to underline that the existing situation is not as it would be, if the needs of older people had been given the attention their scale and nature demand. The proposals in the national service framework do not themselves amount to a strategy, more a commitment to produce one.

Efficiency

In the last 10–15 years successive governments have attempted to make the NHS more efficient as a provider of care, as part of a strategy of trying to contain costs. Applying this criterion to research would imply a focus on areas where costs can be reduced. It is always risky to assert that 'there is no research' in a particular area, but as far as we are aware, no official paper of the last ten years has identified cost containment as a research priority, although it has clearly been a policy priority, and there is no programme of work devoted to it within the ambit of the Department of Health.

PROPOSALS FOR ORGANISATION OF RESEARCH: NATIONAL SERVICE FRAMEWORK FOR OLDER PEOPLE

The Framework states that the research strategy will be implemented through:

- **An advisory network** – advice on developing and implementing this strategy will be taken from scientific experts and researchers in a wide variety of disciplines as well as those using findings of research to improve clinical decisions and service delivery for older people, and users themselves. The strategy will also take account of the burden of disease, potential benefits, policy priorities and the responsibilities and work of other funders.
- **A directed portfolio of research** on older people – the portfolio director will work with the National Director for Services for Older People and take account of research that has implications for older people under existing portfolios.
- **A funders forum on ageing research** – a national forum of key funders of research on health and social care related to older people has been established and will meet twice a year. The forum's overall aim will be to stimulate and facilitate multidisciplinary working and develop research activities across the boundaries between research funders.

(Department of Health, 2001g, para.35)

In fact the need for such research was identified as long ago as the 1950s in the report of the Committee of Enquiry into the Cost of the National Health Service:

> *700. We are of the opinion that the knowledge at present available about the working of the National Health Service is inadequate and should be considerably extended and improved, since it is only on the basis of such knowledge that the right decisions can be made for the future development of the Service. We need to know more, for example, about the economies of hospital management, e.g.*
>
> - *what is the most economical size of a hospital to undertake any specific functions*

- *about the nature and causes of differences of morbidity in different Hospital Regions*
- *about the changing patterns in the use of drugs in the National Health Service, and also about their cost*
- *about the incidence of charges on particular sections of the community (revealing, for example, the extent to which demands have been postponed or abandoned and the effect which this will have on the future pattern of supply)*
- *about the relative costs of institutional and domiciliary treatment, and so on*

Guillebaud, 1956, p.233

It is possible to identify some recent work bearing on most of these areas, but not all. For example, in the last ten years there has been no officially supported original work on the optimum scale of particular hospital functions (Ferguson *et al.*, 1997).

The Audit Commission and to a lesser degree the National Audit Office have carried out a great deal of work relevant to efficiency, and there is a modest amount of academic work (Jenkins-Clarke *et al.*, 1997) on issues such as skill-mix or self-care, both of which are partly driven by the need to contain costs. But, as with ageing, up to the time of the publication of the national service framework, the field lacks commitment: there is no institutional focus for developing and implementing research ideas bearing on the whole field of efficiency in service delivery and cost containment.[36] As a result, when the Treasury determines, as it has done for over a decade, what scale of efficiency improvement the NHS should approve, it can only take a figure out of thin air.

Similarly the inquiry into the future costs of the NHS (Wanless, 2001) had very little substantive work to rely on relating to the scope for raising productivity or achieving efficiency gains. Indeed it was compelled, in its interim report, to ask for evidence on this very issue.

Another approach, given the continuing need to contain costs, would be to focus on particularly expensive diseases. One criterion – used, for example, by the World Health Organisation – is the significance of a particular disease in terms of the cost of treatment and its implications for those suffering it and society as a whole (Murray and Lopez, 1996).

---

36. Harrison and Dixon (2000) proposed quixotically that a Cost Commission should be established to supply such a focus.

This approach – generally known as the burden of disease approach – will inevitably 'favour' the major diseases which are recognised as priorities.[37]

The Department of Health has never attempted to use this approach systematically – although it is one of the criteria referred to in *Research for Health*. There are objections to it both of a practical nature and of an ethical nature if used as the sole criterion for determining which areas should attract funding because of its implications for small need groups. Nevertheless, it clearly makes sense to ensure that 'expensive' diseases attract sustained research attention.

But, as Rothwell has recently argued, this common sense conclusion has not been drawn in the case of stroke:

> *although individual governments and the WHO have highlighted the importance of prevention and treatment of stroke, spending on research is very low, and lags a long way behind heart disease and cancer.*
>
> Rothwell, 2001, p.1612[38]

In taking this condition, we are not seeking to endorse this particular case, but rather to bring out the general point which Rothwell's paper reveals: that there is no publicly available framework within which a case for more spending in this or any other area can be made. The focus on the three national priorities appears to have sidelined any attempt to take a comprehensive view even across the main disease areas.

Organisation and delivery

We have argued elsewhere that the R&D programme has persistently ignored certain types of problem:

> *The continuing emphasis on clinical issues in research priorities means that the issues identified in earlier chapters as critical to the running of the Service remain neglected. This neglect is not simply a*

---

37. See Gross *et al.* (1999), who found that existing allocation of National Institutes of Health funding seem to favour certain conditions and lead to relative neglect of others, but they point out that different ways of measuring the burden of disease produce different 'desirable' allocations of research funds. They also identify a number of other limitations of this approach.

38. Rothwell's paper underlines many of the points made in this study.

matter of lack of resources; rather, it stems from a persistent failure to acknowledge the implications of the central and the local management role, in particular, the vast range of areas where clinical and other issues interrelate and can only be tackled by combining skills and disciplines. In other words, the needs of the NHS as a system of health care delivery have been neglected.

Harrison and Dixon, 2000, p.234

To those working in the area of health services research (or operational research as the 1988 report described it) this conclusion is painfully evident (see, for example, Melzer, 1998). For broad policy areas such as access to elective care and waiting lists or the reconfiguration of hospitals, a trawl through the research register proves extremely disappointing – the result, depending on the precise research terms used, is usually nil. (A search on 'hospital organisation', for example, produces no results.) There is no mention in the reports cited in this and the previous chapter of hospital restructuring or improving access to elective care despite the importance of these to national policy objectives such as waiting time/list targets and the hospital building programme currently being financed largely through the PFI.[39]

In fact the Department of Health *Yearbook of Research and Development 1990* does contain a section on acute services, but the work reported is all focused on particular interventions. None refers to the institution in which the interventions take place or to the circumstances (e.g. scale of activity, mix of locally available specialties) which are likely to impact on how effective they may be in practice. Since then, acute hospitals have not attracted a research programme in their own right.

This gap became evident to all when the then Secretary of State, Frank Dobson, commissioned the National Bed Inquiry in 1998. It found the Department of Health in an intellectual vacuum, short of data, research findings and analytic technique. It should be emphasised that this vacuum existed at departmental level. Many of those working there possessed substantial knowledge of the field, but this was not harnessed as a collective product.[40] Like the Wanless report, the Inquiry raised a

---

39. Research was carried out for the then Department of Health and Social Security during the 1970s which identified the key issues relevant to waiting list research: 25 years later they remain to be addressed.

40. The vacuum is being filled albeit slowly.

series of questions on which it sought evidence, questions such as the right balance between hospital and community facilities, which would have been systematically addressed before if the 'needs of the NHS' had actually commanded the appropriate resources.

The SDO programme represents an attempt to overcome this failure: the list of areas identified through the consultation process it undertook soon after its launch would, if tackled vigorously, lead to a substantial shift in the balance of activity. But by the end of 2001 it had made only a small number of commissions and spending remained very low – much less than the £1 million initially budgeted for 2000/01. Few would contest the areas it has decided to support (see its website, www.sdo.lshtm.ac.uk/ for details), but they do not amount to a substantial attack on how best to improve day-to-day service delivery.

This reflects what Sir Michael Peckham, the first Director of the R&D programme, has termed a deep-rooted bias in favour of R and against D. He has argued in a book published after his retirement from his post as Director of R&D that:

> Research and development is an essential component of the internal mechanisms needed to correct the discrepancy between technological sophistication and organisational dysfunction. However, to be effective it needs to be amplified and complemented by an effective and coherent service development function. The challenge of absorbing and imaginatively exploiting technologies and of implementing and refining new policies constitutes a massive developmental task, yet there is no dedicated capacity within the National Health Service capable of tackling these questions efficiently and responsively.

> Peckham, 1996, p.144

He concluded therefore that 'the requirements for health service development need to be separately defined and supported'. He goes on to note that:

> The development task includes issues related to hospitals and other elements of the health care built environment, health service infrastructure, user and workforce questions, the design of health service processes and delivery systems, and the relationship between lay people and professional staff. The scope of development also encompasses issues such as clinical guidelines, quality and

performance measures, as well as the criteria and mechanisms for medical self-regulation.

Peckham, 1996, p.145

A start has been made with the collaborative programmes into cancer (which refer to local efforts to improve service design and delivery) and the 'action on' series (targeted at particular services to improve care delivery on the ground), but these are essentially tactical in nature. They lack the clout to take on all the issues which Sir Michael identifies, which would involve questioning all the professional roles, including those of managers and senior clinicians.

Furthermore, there are signs in the consultation papers that a fundamental point has yet to be grasped. The King's Fund response (Harrison and Mulligan, 2000) to the consultation paper *NHS Priorities and Needs Funding* (Department of Health, 2000e) argued the paper had not attempted to define the 'needs of the NHS' in a systematic way:

> *Implicit in the paper is the disaggregated tradition of medical science and clinical practice which focuses on sharply defined problems within particular services or particular clinical conditions. As a consequence, it does not explicitly acknowledge issues which run right across the whole Service, or broad parts of it, nor those which span the Service and other fields of public policy.*

These issues, of which hospital building and reconfiguration are prime examples, require the assembly of a large amount of disparate knowledge. Here the need is for intelligence gathering and synthesis and the bringing together of knowledge and expertise from a broad range of disciplines. Work of this kind bearing on hospitals was commissioned from the University of York (Ferguson *et al.*, 1997), but this exercise has been one-off: there is no continuing focus on this area.

This gap has been partially filled by the Foresight programme run by the Office of Science and Technology. This has produced a number of reports bearing on health. The most recent (DTI/OST, 2001c)[41] argued for a systematic analysis of current and likely future trends comprising a searching appraisal of the design and organisation of the next generation

---

41. See also the earlier Foresight report (DTI/OST, 1995) which emphasises, e.g. in respect of ageing, the need to integrate across disciplines and existing research centres.

of hospitals which would define the range of tasks to be performed in them, bearing in mind technological, health and other trends. To do this would require expertise:

> in such areas as spatial analysis, transportation, architecture, bioengineering and health technologies, systems, human behaviour, informatics and have input from medical and other professional staff.

DTI/OST, 2001c, p.9

But where is such a conjunction of expertise to be found? A recent study on the future of the hospital points out that:

> Presently there is a lack of a single source of knowledge to guide important decisions, e.g. by staff planning PFI hospitals. We need to reuse existing knowledge and lessons and place timely best practice information within easy reach of both health service clients and designers in a national information exchange dedicated to health care design and construction. Post occupancy evaluation could provide valuable feedback on performance for future development.

Francis and Glanville, 2001

It therefore recommends that there should be: 'a forum for exploring new ideas' which would look at topics such as:

> the implications of managed clinical networks, reconfiguration, digital technologies, and the bringing together of design quality, sustainability with modularisation of the built environment.

Francis and Glanville, 2001, p.156

The need for these proposals stems directly from the fact that the areas covered in these reports has not been satisfactorily addressed in existing research programmes, nor does a suitable institution exist to promote research in them. In other words, the supply side of the research economy has to be addressed if needs such as these are to be met. However the main reason that the supply side of the health research economy has not developed in these areas stems from a persistent failure for the demand side to develop for major projects of this kind.[42] The following chapter looks further into this 'chicken-and-egg' problem.

---

42. In April 2001 the formation of a Department of Health-led process on hospital restructuring was announced.

Determining priorities

The 1993 report *Research for Health* refers to:

> *a systematic approach to identifying and setting R&D priorities, in which NHS staff and the users of the Service are being asked to identify important issues which confront them and, in partnership with the research community, to characterise and prioritise these problems as the basis for seeking solutions.*

Department of Health, 1993b

It goes on to elaborate what 'systematic' is intended to mean in practice, including a number of relevant criteria such as burden of disease to the NHS and the community, prevalence, policy priorities, feasibility of research and potential benefits. It also notes that small groups should not be left out of consideration.

Nevertheless, in 1994 the Culyer Task Force recommended that:

> *the NHS should make explicit the basis on which decisions on its investment in R&D and service support for R&D will be taken at both national and local levels. We recommend that the NHS should develop and publish the principles and criteria which will guide the use at national level and local levels of NHS funds related to R&D.*

Culyer, 1994a, para.9

This recommendation has not been systematically addressed, although, as the box on HTA (p.109) shows, the HTA programme has set out an explicit and systematic process in summary form. Recent policy statements refer to the national priorities where targets for health improvement have been set. They do not reflect a sustained attempt to consider 'the needs of the NHS' across the whole field.[43]

Recent papers acknowledge that the process for determining the allocation of research resources is far from being fully developed. 'Next Steps' states that:

> *The long term aim is strategic coherence across the whole of NHS R&D.*

---

43. This gap has in part been filled by the Foresight programme, particularly in its recent report *Health 2020* on which we have already drawn. However, the impetus behind this programme comes from the Department of Trade and Industry rather than the Department of Health.

and adds that:

> *The key task in the next two years is to take stock of all NHS R&D that*
> *does not have an eligible external funder and organise it into coherent*
> *programmes that are consistent with the emerging operational*
> *principles for NHS Priorities and Needs R&D Funding.*

Department of Health, 2001l, para.5.2

Furthermore, a Department of Health position paper issued in 2001 states
that:

> *5.5 Strategic reviews will comprise:*
>
> ■ *assessment of national public health and service priorities for that*
>   *topic*
> ■ *assessment of the needs for new knowledge arising from these*
>   *priorities*
> ■ *expert review of the balance of current research activity compared*
>   *with these needs*
> ■ *decisions on future NHS R&D priorities*
> ■ *communication of priorities, and planning to deliver results across*
>   *them.*

Department of Health, 2001f, p.15

These very general aims in themselves embody an admission that little
progress has been made towards achieving a mix of projects which
promise to make the best possible contribution to promoting the nation's
health. This is not to suggest that there is some simple formula which
the Department could apply to identify such a mix. But statements about
the process of defining a process do not represent progress towards
tackling the very difficult issues which selection of the 'best' mix
presents.

User involvement in determining priorities

In 1995, a Standing Advisory Group on Consumer Involvement in the
NHS R&D programme was established. Its first report found 'important
mismatches between professional and consumer views' (NHS Executive,
1998, para.7.6). Two years later the strategic review of the levy
recommended that 'all health services research should involve
consumers of health services at every stage in the research process'.

As a result, users are now represented on most if not all groups considering research needs. These developments, while welcome, are only a beginning and their impact on what research projects are selected for support has not been evaluated.

Health service users are of course the ultimate customers for health-related research. As we noted in Chapter 3, the central perception of the Rothschild report was that there was no informed customer for the research then being carried out by the MRC and its recommendations were designed to encourage the Department of Health and Social Security to take on that role. But as far as the NHS is concerned, the Department could only be a 'proxy' customer and the same is true of the NHS. If, as the cliché has it, 'services are for patients', then so should be the research programme which aims to improve the services.

According to Tallon and colleagues:

> We have noted a clear mismatch between the interventions that are researched, and those regularly used and prioritised by consumers. The results of our focus group and survey shows that people use various treatment options and want information on all these, and that professional groups want high-quality evidence for all interventions. However, the review of published and unpublished studies shows a massive concentration of research in drug and surgical treatments. This finding suggests a need to broaden the research agenda to investigate whether other treatments are as effective as drug and surgical interventions.
>
> Tallon et al., 2000, p.2039

This conclusion poses a substantial challenge to the way the health research economy now works. It is not just a matter of this project rather than that, or even this disease rather than that, but of a deep-seated provider-led bias into certain kinds of treatment, treatments which users may prefer to avoid if there are options available. To a degree, those seeking help from alternative therapies (whether effective or not) are 'voting' for forms of treatment which mainstream services do not embody.

The issue arises even with mainstream services. As we have shown else-where (Harrison, 2001), some of the fundamental features of the delivery of health care such as the structure of specialisms stem from professional debates almost unheeded by health policy, still less research.[44] But the wider availability of information and other forces are changing the relationship between professional and user, though the process of thinking through what that actually means has been slow to develop.[45]

Progress has been made, however, in involving a wider range of people in the process of determining what areas should be researched and what projects should be supported in those parts of the Department of Health/NHS programme which have a coherent organisation. The many committees set up to carry out topic reviews have allowed more 'voices' to be heard. More specifically, the HTA programme embodies a highly organised and explicit process of determining which projects it should support. HTA is conducted in a way which is self-consciously 'open': its website invites users to make suggestions on research areas and to contribute to the programme; it also sets out activities designed to involve users. Similarly, soon after its establishment, SDO conducted an extensive 'listening exercise' within the NHS and elsewhere (see boxes on SDO and HTA, overleaf).

As is now recognised in the NHS Plan and the more recent *Expert Patient* paper (Department of Health, 2001k), taking users seriously requires research into how they want services to be delivered and the redesign of services in the light of that information. But the logic of this process has yet to be extended to determining what research programmes would be required to underpin radical service design around patients' views, taking a 'zero-base' view of current professional roles and procedures, i.e. a genuinely strategic approach. How to do this is worth substantial research in its own right.

---

44. There is a literature, largely American, on the origin of specialties, but very little work looking at the question normatively. See, for example, Stevens (1998).

 45. See www.conres.co.uk for a recent overview and links to relevant sites.

THE SDO PROGRAMME

When the SDO programme was formally launched in 2000, an extensive 'listening exercise' was conducted resulting in the identification of ten areas of concern:

- organising health services around the needs of the patient
- user involvement
- continuity of care
- co-ordination/integration across organisations
- inter-professional working
- workforce issues
- relationship between organisational form, function and outcomes
- implications of the communication revolution
- use of resources, such as ways of disinvesting in services and managing demand
- implementation of major national policy initiatives such as the national service frameworks for coronary heart disease and mental health.

The early work commissioned by the SDO programme reflects some of the above. This work includes, for example, a systematic review of continuity of care.

The lack of a set of principles to guide allocation

Chapter 2 defined a number of roles for the State – in this case primarily the Department of Health – and in this way defined in general terms what the contribution of publicly funded programmes should be. But neither the Department of Health nor organisations sponsored by it such as the CRDC have attempted to set out any general philosophy or set of principles to guide the overall allocation of resources.[46] Nor have they, our examples suggest, been able to ensure that major areas where there are indisputable research needs have received sustained attention.

---

46. See Institute of Medicine (1998) for an attempt to do this in the USA.

DETERMINING PRIORITIES WITHIN THE HTA PROGRAMME

According to the HTA programme's website, 'Effective prioritisation lies at the heart of the Health Technology Assessment (HTA) Programme. It involves choosing which of the many suggestions received … should become one of the 40 or so which will become commissioned research each year.'

The programme is supported by the 50 or so members of three advisory panels. These cover:

- diagnostic technologies and screening
- pharmaceuticals
- therapeutic procedures.

Panel members have a wide range of backgrounds and bring considerable experience and expertise. Consumers attend the advisory panel meetings as voting members. In addition, some 180 experts working in the NHS research community provide advice on specific topics.

The website describes the process in some detail, but the main points are these:

- All the suggestions received by the HTA programme are considered and great care is taken to ensure that they are prioritised appropriately. The process of deciding which of the suggestions become 'priorities' is a crucial element of the programme and is central to its success. The panels discuss suggestions before deciding, by ballot, which should be taken forward.
- Panel members pay particular attention to the burden of the health problem and its cost, the degree of current uncertainty and the urgency and cost of the research. Few of the suggestions originally submitted survive this rigorous scrutiny as topics are prioritised.
- The National Co-ordinating Centre for HTA then prepares briefing papers ('vignettes') on those suggestions which remain. The vignette brings much more detail to the proposal by clarifying the research question and the extent of the health problem. This allows the advisory panel, at a later meeting, to give the proposal more informed consideration. Each panel examines about 15 vignettes each year.

As far as the first of these is concerned, the Department of Health R&D website simply states:

> *priorities take account of widespread consultation with those using, delivering and managing services within a framework overseen by the Central Research & Development Committee for the NHS. Priorities reflect analysis of the burden of disease, potential benefits, Government priorities and take account of the responsibilities and work of other funders.*

This brief and in itself uncontentious statement had not, at the time of writing, been elaborated into a systematic statement of principles, of explicit justification of the current allocation of resources or of plans to change that allocation. Our overall conclusion must therefore be that a systematic way of defining the 'best possible' allocation of research resources within the control of the Department of Health remains to be found.[47]

Overview

The processes we have briefly described in the first part of this chapter can be seen as a response to one of the central criticisms made by the House of Lords Committee: that the then pattern of publicly funded research was overly influenced by the providers of research rather than its users. The various subject area committees, and the HTA programme in particular, have engaged large numbers of research users in the process of determining what should be funded. In that sense, the process has become much more pluralistic: a larger range of 'voices' can make themselves heard, including those of research users and health service users. This is a considerable advance on the situation described in the 1988 report.

However, the 'gap claims' set out above suggest that the current pattern of spending continues to embody significant biases of a kind identified in 1988. In part this shortfall stems from the inherent difficulty of prioritising research across the very broad fields of interest that the Department of Health is responsible for. The nature of the gains to be achieved in

---

47. See Working Group on Priority Setting (1997) and Institute of Medicine (1998) for a lengthy discussion of how research priorities are determined within the US public sector.

different areas is that they are incommensurate and, while there has been limited progress in determining the value of research which has already been carried out and in determining the possible value of proposed research, these methods are not sufficiently advanced to be generally deployed.

But in part it is due to a more fundamental failure to take stock of the whole field in which the Department of Health has a role or in which, because of the wider public health agenda, an interest. Lacking a general set of principles to guide the allocation of resources, the Department of Health cannot make systematic decisions about what it funds, or fully justify the decisions it does make. Implicitly the Department of Health is claiming the so-called priority areas – cancer, mental health and coronary heart disease – have greater priority than all others, but these claims have been asserted rather than demonstrated. Moreover, as we shall see in Chapter 7, even within a priority area such as cancer, claims for the existence of gaps and bias against certain kinds of research can be plausibly made.

With a general set of principles to guide the allocation of research funds, the Department of Health would be in a position to address the biases which are implicit in the current pattern of spending – biases which lead to the neglect of some areas almost entirely both within the publicly funded part of the health research economy and within the economy as a whole. We develop the latter point in Chapter 6. Before doing so we look at the other half of the health research economy, the providers.

Chapter 5

The supply of research

In some fields the supply of health research has been weak and has been unable to expand to meet increased demand. This chapter examines longstanding barriers to developing research capacity at the level of the individual, the profession or area of research and the institutions in which research takes place.

5 The supply of research

The health research economy sketched out in Chapter 1 can and does respond, like any other part of the economy, to changes in demand. Since the time of the 1988 report, it has expanded enormously – primarily due to the growth of private for-profit research, but also due to a sustained if modest increase within the public sector. Nevertheless, the supply side of the research economy has been seen as problematic ever since attempts were made to develop publicly funded research outside the ambit of the MRC.

In most markets, it can be assumed with some confidence that if the demand is there, the supply will be forthcoming (with some obvious exceptions such as land). In the case of publicly financed health-related research, that assumption does not hold. The 1988 Committee found that, in areas such as nursing and other non-medical professions, the provider side was weak and entry to it hard to negotiate. Because of lack of suitable provision, gaps recognised by payers or commissioners could not – and still cannot – be filled.

Suitable provision cannot emerge without sustained demand. No organisation, public or private, can afford to invest in the process of creating research capacity, which is necessarily a long-term affair, without a clear prospect of there being demand to use it once it is in place. But no funding agency will commit large amounts of cash when there is only limited prospect of it being used productively.

This 'chicken-and-egg' problem bears on individual researchers. If they wish to work in certain kinds of health-related research, particularly if they work in areas which, unlike medicine, do not have a long research tradition, there is no clear career structure for them. Without that, many are deterred from entry or leave early for securer working environments. It also bears on professions and institutions. Professions without a research tradition need to demonstrate that they can use funds well – but they cannot do that without a track record. Some research requires large resources and the ability to put together teams from a number of disciplines. The universities by their nature are potentially 'in the market' for such work, but the effort of creating new forms of organisation or new academic grouping will not appear worthwhile unless a substantial commitment of funds is in prospect.

This chapter looks at the supply side of the health research economy in three stages:

- the individual
- the profession or area of research
- the organisation or institution.

It then goes on to outline the policy responses to a series of reports which have identified, time and again, the same weaknesses in the system.

As in previous chapters, the House of Lords 1988 report provides our starting point.

Individuals

The 1988 report found that while 'research rests on the availability of well-qualified and talented researchers':

> *Many witnesses fear that research workers are not being recruited and trained in the United Kingdom in sufficient numbers, and that career prospects are not attractive enough to keep researchers in the medical field in this country. The Committee are persuaded that this is the case. Poor pay and poor career prospects are both serious disincentives. It is not uncommon for a post-graduate research post to be advertised at a salary lower than would be paid to a typist in many other fields, and moreover such posts are normally in short-term contracts providing no career prospects whatever. Training grants are very low. These failings have to be remedied.*

It therefore concluded that:

> *Policies to ensure that researchers and their supporting staff are available in the right fields are integral to the setting of priorities in medical research.*

> House of Lords, 1988, para.5.17

In its response to the report, the Government accepted 'that the career progression of those engaged in research, especially clinical research, should be taken into account in decisions on NHS manpower policy' (Department of Health, 1989, para.31.3). But this commitment probably meant less than it appeared to. NHS manpower policy could scarcely be relied on to solve a problem that affected, in the context of the NHS, only a small group of people. Workforce planning was not well developed at the time, and there were difficulties in matching training to 'the needs of the Service' even to meet well-established needs, such as for extra doctors. The response was, therefore, a response in name only, nor did the Government commitment mean anything for those seeking careers in universities. Not surprisingly, the problem continued to be identified in successive reports.

In 1992, a review of the research units funded by the Department of Health found that, even though many had been in existence for many years and their funding was on a six-year rolling basis, most staff were on project contracts of a shorter term and 'because good research staff cannot personally afford to remain on short-term contracts, they move out of research' (Department of Health, 1992, para.40).

The Culyer Task Force also found that the supply of research was problematic:

> 3.109 *We were told of the lack of career paths and incentives for some researchers and for others working in the R&D field within the NHS, particularly the non-clinical professions. We have also heard of the preponderance of short term contracts for research staff. These appear to us potentially important disincentives to attracting and retaining people needed to carry out R&D within the NHS. Without further development of appropriate career structures and incentives for researchers and R&D support staff there may not be enough trained researchers in the future. That development would have to take into account the additional problems stemming from the need for increased mobility of researchers as R&D moves into primary and community care.*
>
> Culyer, 1994a

The Task Force therefore recommended:

> *developing a human resource strategy for R&D in the NHS, embracing training and more general personnel issues.*
>
> Culyer, 1994a, p.50

In 1995, the results of a study commissioned from Social and Community Planning Research (SCPR) by the Department of Health and the NHS Executive into research workforce capacity were published (Lewis and Ritchie, 1995). This extensive review acknowledged that 'the environment for health and social care research was ... improving' but its findings also reinforced those of the Task Force: career prospects were found to be poor, as was the status of those engaged in this kind of research.

In 1996 the Department of Health issued a 'First Statement of a Research Capacity Strategy' (Department of Health, 1996a) following a commitment made in its response to the House of Lords 1995 report. In its foreword, this acknowledged 'the scale and difficulty of the issues that now need to be addressed' and it set out a large number of areas where improvements were required.

Subsequently, the strategic review of the levy concluded:

> *25. A major weakness in the present Research & Development programme is the shortage of experienced health service researchers in a well developed career structure. This shortage is a major threat to the Research & Development programme.*
>
> Department of Health, 1999a

The lack of career structures and the other weaknesses referred to in the box opposite clearly stem from the context in which research is carried out. The SCPR study pointed to changes in the funding which were inimical to the development of research skills:

> *The emphasis of the [research] programmes was seen to be shifting from theoretical, basic, long term research to applied, evaluative, short term research. ... The limited availability of long term funding was seen to impede the ability of research teams and individuals to build expertise in specialist areas.*
>
> Lewis and Ritchie, 1995, p.2

The weakness also makes it hard for institutions to provide for long-term careers, and it is at this level that solutions have to be found. Before

WEAKNESSES IDENTIFIED IN CAREERS IN RESEARCH

The difficulties facing individuals are common to other areas of research. Despite the importance successive governments have attached to the UK's science base, there is widespread failure to recognise scientific research as a profession in its own right. A paper from the Association of Researchers in Medicine and Science concludes that:

> *The present structure of research organisation is **obsolete and requires review**. In particular, given that the most important element in any research enterprise is the human resource, the outmoded practice of recruitment, training and employment of research workers has become increasingly inadequate in the current climate of scientific and technological endeavour.*

It therefore proposes that:

- *research (academic) institutions should extend their **contractual responsibility** for the management and funding of research projects or programmes; and*
- *research institutions should establish **career grade research posts** as the core of their research base.*

The paper sets out the weaknesses of the existing system as follows:

> a) *Able young persons are clearly discouraged from seeking employment where there is no adequate career structure or reasonable perceived expectation of advancement, and where the system is loaded against increasing age and experience.*
> b) *Considerable resources are wasted in the training of highly skilled individuals who may be lost from research altogether and may be difficult to re-deploy by the age at which they become surplus to the capacity of a poorly managed system.*
> c) *Poor prospects, as much as poor financial rewards, have resulted in a significant loss of talent to our industrial and intellectual competitors in the EC and USA.*
> d) *The failure to attract high calibre individuals and train them in research techniques and skills is a serious loss to industries requiring expertise to maintain their lead in a modern technological environment.*

continued overleaf

WEAKNESSES IDENTIFIED IN CAREERS IN RESEARCH *continued*

e) *The reliance on fixed term contracts for the funding of research staff leads to a widespread requirement to promote projects with short-term objectives.*

f) *Inefficiency caused by: i) time lost by the contract researcher looking for the next contract post; ii) the researcher leaving before the end of the contract; iii) the difficulty of finding suitably qualified researchers to undertake projects that are either short-term by design, or have only a short period to run because the previous researcher left.*

g) *Bias against employment of female staff because of difficulties in 'f' above arising in respect of maternity leave, or career breaks.*

ARMS, 2001, pp.2–5

Although not a response to the above, the Department of Trade and Industry white paper *Excellence and Opportunity* expresses concern 'about career development prospects for young people starting out' in research careers (DTI, 2000b, para.34). Since then the Roberts (2002) report has proposed a series of measures designed to improve career prospects across the science base as a whole.

considering these however we look at the second area of 'supply failure', professions or fields of expertise.

Professions and fields

The 1988 report concluded that areas such as nursing, dentistry and professions allied to medicine were 'being marginalised in the setting of national priorities for research' (House of Lords, 1988, para.4.10).

Nursing

A review of research in nursing midwifery and health visiting published in 1993 (Department of Health, 1993a) noted that the Department had begun commissioning nursing research in 1968 and it remained the principal source of funding. But it also found that a majority of the projects in research databases were carried out by individuals in their own time – scarcely an indication of a substantial commitment of public funds. Rafferty and Traynor (1998) found some years later that the same situation persisted: only one-third of the nursing research papers they identified acknowledged a funding source.[48]

The central conclusion of the 1993 Department of Health report was that:

> *The overriding need is for a substantial and robust body of health services research – and within it, of research in nursing – to set alongside the illustrious tradition of basic clinical bio-medical research.*

> Department of Health, 1993a, para.2.2.2

To this end it made a series of recommendations designed to offset the imbalance, in particular:

> *that the professional organisations in association with those charitable organisations currently supporting research in nursing, establish a coherent and effective means of reviewing their research needs, monitoring progress and contributing to the formulation of research agenda at national and regional levels.*

> Department of Health, 1993a, para.3.49

In 1997 the decision to appoint a professor of nursing to lead nursing research policy was announced. Subsequently David Thompson was appointed to:

- set up an advisory committee on priorities for nursing, midwifery and health visiting research
- advise on how nurses could be encouraged to contribute to and make use of research evidence
- work with the research workforce development group.

(Department of Health, 1997a)

Two years later, a Department of Health paper on the role of nursing and other professions within the NHS recognised the need for R&D

---

48. See also Payne (1993) who reports a study of nursing research projects in cancer care. Of the ten identified, eight were for higher degrees and the majority were only partially funded. 'Moreover, eight of the ten projects were being undertaken to fulfil the requirements of a higher degree. This implies that the researchers were relatively inexperienced' (p.117).

(Department of Health 1999i). This was followed in 2000 by *Towards a Strategy for Nursing Research and Development* which acknowledges that:

> *Despite considerable progress in recent years current arrangements fail to maximise the nursing contribution to research and development. Some constraints are self-imposed ... but nurses have also encountered institutionalised barriers that have constrained development of both capacity and capability.*

Department of Health, 2000a, para.3

TOWARDS A STRATEGY FOR NURSING RESEARCH AND DEVELOPMENT

This paper makes a series of proposals designed to redress the weaknesses it identified, including the following:

- It is recommended that the Research and Development Workforce Capacity Implementation Group should be asked to undertake or commission work to establish current capacity to address nursing issues in the priority areas for Department of Health/NHS research, and how best to address deficiencies.
- It is recommended that the Research and Development Workforce Capacity Implementation Group be asked to develop proposals to pilot new and innovative career paths and to explore and publicise how best to maximise investment funded by NHS education and training levies, and other funding sources, to build research capacity.
- It is recommended that the Department of Health should establish a time-limited initiative of pre and post-doctoral research training fellowships and career scientist awards.
- It is recommended that the Department of Health should explore with the Higher Education Funding Council for England and with other funding bodies the potential for greater co-operation and coherence of investment.
- It is recommended that the Department of Health explore options for pump-priming a handful of designated centres with thematic research and development programmes to help build capacity through partnerships and collaboration, focusing on links with the NHS and service delivery.

(Department of Health, 2000a, pp.4–6)

It goes on:

> *In simplistic terms, a vicious circle militates against a full and active nursing contribution.*

Department of Health, 2000a, para.4

Development of nursing research

Rafferty and Traynor (2000) used an analysis by the Wellcome Trust, *Mapping the Landscape* (Dawson *et al.*, 1998), to track the progress of nursing research. This indicates that the nursing field has been growing rapidly, but from a low base.

TABLE 6: BIOMEDICAL SUBFIELDS RANKED BY NUMBER OF UK PUBLICATIONS, 1988–95, WITH AVERAGE ANNUAL PERCENTAGE GROWTH (AAPG)		
SUBFIELD	No.	AAPG
Neurosciences	25,240	3.7
Genetics	20,620	9.3
Oncology	19,654	4.5
Cardiology	19,084	4.3
Immunology	17,186	1.8
Gastroenterology	14,945	1.8
Obstetrics and gynaecology	12,069	3.4
Respiratory medicine	9,969	4.5
Histopathology	8,682	1.9
Arthritis and rheumatism	6,672	6.0
Anaesthesia	6,426	1.4
Developmental biology	6,190	5.1
Ophthalmology	5,354	3.5
Renal medicine	4,660	1.7
Tropical medicine	4,324	3.6
Neonatology	3,989	5.8
Gerontology	3,728	5.0
Nursing research	2,583	15.0
Multiple sclerosis	725	3.6

This brief history suggests that the obstacles to the development of an effective supply side are numerous and substantial.[49] Report after report has identified essentially the same obstacles. As we now show, however, they are not confined to nursing.

Primary care

It was recognised in the early 1990s that, paralleling changes in service delivery, the balance of research should switch to community settings. The Culyer levy made that feasible and some degree of reallocation of research funding resulted. Subsequently the primary care white paper *Delivering the Future* (Department of Health, 1996a) proposed that research spending in this area should be increased from £25 million to £50 million. The £50 million target was confirmed in 1997 by the Health Minister, Alan Milburn, when announcing the Government's response to the national working group report on R&D in primary care.

In 1996 the CRDC set up a national working group to carry out a strategic review of R&D in primary care. The subsequent report argued the case for an expansion of research in this area and made a large number of recommendations designed to support this objective (NHS Executive, 1997). On its publication, the Department of Health announced three new measures (Department of Health, 1997b) of which the second and third (new training awards and a new regional research network) were directed at improving the supply of research in primary care. But there was no direct response to the funding issue identified in the 1997 report which had concluded that:

> *The new funding arrangements for NHS Providers are not the most appropriate mechanism for developing primary care R&D capacity in situations where it does not presently exist. Such development should be supported through the NHS R&D Programme.*

> NHS Executive, 1997, p.49

In the same year the MRC published a topic review *Primary Health Care*

---

49. Rafferty and Traynor (2000) analyse these in detail. Their analysis is too extensive to cite here, but perhaps their central finding lies in the tension they discovered between 'a desire for academic credibility within higher education and for clinical and professional credibility with the local NHS providers' (p.37), a point we look at further in the next chapter.

which considered what had to be done to develop primary care research capacity. It argued that the focus should be on:

- *increasing the supply of principal investigators (non-clinical and clinical)*
- *developing the infrastructure for primary care research*
- *ensuring that those responsible for education in primary care are research-aware, and can apply research evidence to practice*
- *articulating the primary care research perspective.*

MRC, 1997, pp.63–64

A second Department of Health report on research in primary care (Department of Health, 1999g) endorsed many of the 1997 report's findings, but went on to criticise the new funding mechanisms for not providing the support required to build up research capacity:

The initial national programme approach to ... funding was project based but allowed some development and continuity through the length of the programme and the system of dedicated programme management. The move to the new generic funding system may have been increased allocative equity (it is not restricted to specific programmes) but the prioritisation system is cumbersome and unstable and the length of funding too short to allow the development of coherent high quality research. It seems a matter of chance whether a team can go on to do the obvious valuable study implied by the previous one. Emerging groups supported mainly by NHS R&D project funding are very unstable and research expertise is being lost.

Department of Health, 1999g

It therefore went on to recommend that:

Research priorities should be defined to reflect issues of enduring importance to the NHS on a 10–15 year timescale.

The proportion of funding for primary care research which is long term should be increased to achieve institutional stability, encourage continuity of research, and support the development of research expertise.

Department of Health, 1999g

A selection of the report's recommendations bearing on the need for inter-professional work in the field of primary care is shown in the box below.

PRIMARY CARE RESEARCH: SELECTED RECOMMENDATIONS

Recommendation 11. DRD nationally, and RDRDs regionally, should initiate discussion with universities to agree a strategy to ensure that the few established researchers from nursing, health visiting, midwifery, pharmacy, dentistry, optometry and the professions allied to medicine working in primary care are able to develop and consolidate their research skills, particularly in order to support and mentor the next generation of researchers.

Recommendation 12. The NHS Executive should address the current disincentives in career security and salary which discourage primary care clinical staff from following a career in R&D, and from moving between service, teaching and research posts.

Recommendation 13. Separate national support arrangements for optometry, community pharmacy, community midwifery and dentistry should be considered.

Recommendation 14. Most primary care groups (PCGs) will have at least one practice actively involved in research. Such PCGs will need to develop a strategy for supporting and developing research and meeting service costs. It is suggested that responsibility for this strategy is held at board level.

(Department of Health, 1999g)

The 1997 report found that primary care research was largely focused on general practice even though within primary care the prescribing of drugs represents the major cost item and drugs represent the main form of active treatment for patients. In the mid-1990s the Royal Pharmaceutical Society, which is both the regulator and the professional body for pharmacy, began a process of thinking through the future role of pharmacy and the consequent research agenda. A task force reporting in 1997 found that the existing situation was not conducive to good research:

> 78. The Task Force was repeatedly presented with evidence of poor quality in pharmacy practice research, to an extent which would appear

*to indicate problems greater than simply a typical distribution of
human activity. This evidence should not be taken as a reflection of the
individual abilities of the researchers engaged in [pharmacy practice
research] – it is much more the product of the structural and
organisational problems discussed below.*

Royal Pharmaceutical Society of Great Britain, 1997, p.22

It then went on to point to a series of methodological weaknesses:

- *very few evaluative studies had been undertaken, and those that
  were published were often based on single sites and poorly
  controlled for bias*
- *data collection was often undertaken by the pharmacist providing
  the service*
- *the objectivity of the researcher was often undermined by extrinsic
  concerns (e.g. the need to justify a proposed service development)*
- *sample sizes were often too small, and response rates poor*
- *little or no attempt was made to establish the impact which non-
  responders might have had on the findings*
- *little attempt was made to develop meaningful outcome measures.*

Royal Pharmaceutical Society of Great Britain, 1997, pp.23–24

This report contained a large number of recommendations for action,
many bearing on the supply of research. These included the formation of
research networks to help organise the work of practice-based
researchers, and the development of research careers and training. It also
contained many recommendations to deal with the need for research
infrastructure within pharmacy research including changes in the use of
NHS levy funding. There has so far been no substantial national-level
response, despite increasing recognition in official papers of the value of
good pharmaceutical advice to both patients and professionals
(Department of Health, 2000f).

Public health

The need for more research into public health was recognised in the 1988
report. The publication of *The Health of the Nation* in 1991 was welcomed
at the time as marking a sea change in policy – moving the NHS away
from the concept of a national sickness service.[50] *A Research and*

---

50. This point had been strongly argued in the Reith Lectures by Kennedy (1981).

Development Strategy for Public Health (Department of Health 2001c) sets out in broad terms a demanding agenda designed to support the promotion of health. This notes that the supply side is not adequate to meet the challenges defined:

> *Although the academic community displays intellectual richness and variety, it is clear that its capacity is insufficient for the scale of the research effort needed. [The Department of Health], in partnership with other main funders, will promote the development of an appropriately skilled and sized workforce for public health R&D.*

Department of Health, 2001c, p.6

The paper points to a large number of practical obstacles to improvement:

> *Issues which need to be addressed include: the lack of career structure in many areas of public health; the difficulty in maintaining and motivating a workforce which has little job security and in which the main funding sources, linked as they are to projects rather than people, may be discontinuous; and the tension between enabling a broad view of public health and participation in R&D for public health, whilst allowing sufficient focus and specialisation to encourage academic excellence.*

Department of Health, 2001c, p.22

In effect this amounts, more than a decade later, to a restatement of the 1988 report findings.

Surgery

Surgery does not lack for prestige within the NHS, but it is essentially a practical, literally hands-on, discipline unsupported by a 'backroom' of laboratory research. A symposium organised by the Office of Health Economics in 1997 set out a wide range of issues bearing on surgical research. The starting point for the symposium was the perception that there was no research culture within surgery. The contributors make it clear that there is not a single problem or answer, but rather a range of factors which make surgical research difficult to organise. These range from the characteristics of surgeons themselves, through the institutions they work in, to relationships with the private sector suppliers of new equipment.

To improve matters, the symposium concluded, requires action on a broad front:

> *The organisation and delivery of R&D is an academic discipline in its own right. It requires rigorous thinking, recognition of the fundamental importance of strategy, and tactical implementation. Applying these principles allows the welding together of teams and the reality of cultural transformation.*

> *the Department of Health, the Royal College of Surgeons, individual specialties, Regional Offices of the NHS Executive and other institutions all have responsibilities for achieving this. A concerted effort is needed to foster an effective R&D culture, including the very important debate about the stature, the credibility and the rewards of surgery in relation to research.*

> Johnston and Sussex, 2000, p.73

Signs of such concerted action are not yet apparent within the Department of Health R&D programme.

Organisations

The NHS inherited a set of teaching/research hospitals which provided the organisational structure, physical facilities and access to patients required for both publicly funded and privately funded research. These institutions continue to dominate the research carried out within the NHS. These centrepieces of the health research economy survived the threat posed by the introduction of the 1990 reforms, and the changes introduced since have not seriously undermined their central position. Nevertheless, their situation within the health research economy remains problematic.

Despite their central importance to the execution of research within the NHS, research hospitals are faced with a dilemma. As a recent study by the Nuffield Trust indicates, they are finding it hard to align the different elements they comprise:

> *NHS Trusts and universities are separately accountable and have differing priorities; they have struggled to manage the paradox of interdependence as independent organisations. The NHS is predominantly focused on service, whereas in universities the*

*priorities are research and education. The changes in the external
environment outlined above have created incentives for organisations
to pursue strategies that point in different directions. There are at
present very few incentives to align research, education and clinical
service strategies.*

Nuffield Trust, 2000, pp.21–22

We will look at these issues in more detail in the next chapter. Suffice to
say here that, despite this failure to make research hospitals coherent
institutions, they do nevertheless by their very existence overcome some
of the supply-side obstacles to the development of research programmes
identified above for other parts of the NHS, embodying as they do
tradition, facilities and organisation.

In contrast to hospitals, other parts of the health research economy have
never enjoyed such a clear and enduring organisational and physical
focus. In principle, the research hospitals could have become the focus of
wider research networks. But the deep-seated divide between hospital
and community put paid to that. A parallel division between medical and
other research has also meant that most resources remain devoted to
areas which impinge on medical practice rather than the work of other
professions and, within medical practice, that part carried out within
the hospital.

Because of their lack of a strong institutional base, community-based
services have not formed part of the science base. The consultation paper
setting out how the science base element of funding should work
acknowledged this weakness, stating that 'The Department of Health is
committed to developing R&D in primary care and is developing
arrangements to ensure the most appropriate access to NHS Support for
Science in the primary care sector' (Department of Health, 2000g,
para.2.5). It goes on to state (para.2.6.1) the intention that GPs and other
contractors will have access on an equivalent basis to trusts. But this
does not deal with the lack of an institutional base comparable to a
hospital.

Successive reviews of primary care research have put forward proposals
designed to overcome this. The 1997 review of primary care discussed at
some length the notion of networks which would facilitate and encourage
collaborative R&D and also discussed supporting GPs in conducting their
own R&D (NHS Executive, 1997).

Subsequently, the notion of a community teaching trust was floated (Jackson, 2001). This would:

■ provide an alternative and attractive 'portfolio' career option for GPs and other primary and community health care professionals
■ increase the number of high-quality GPs, nurses and other primary and community care staff, especially in areas which have traditionally found it difficult to recruit
■ develop the skills of health and social care staff
■ use enhanced skills to further develop the provision of primary and community care services
■ provide a learning and resource centre for dissemination of good practice and learning across a local health care system.

At present neither the notion of networks nor the notion of a community teaching trust has got fully off the ground. Hence the development of a proper organisational basis for research in the community-based professions paralleling the research hospital has only just begun.

However, as we have argued elsewhere (Harrison, 2001), the emphasis in thinking about how health is delivered should be on systems of care rather than professions or organisations. In this context, the still-prevailing primary/secondary/tertiary distinctions are irrelevant and misleading. Rather, health care delivery should be seen as a series of pathways clustered into systems of care which run across all health providers. This view is slowly becoming the conventional one and its implications for research recognised.

The mental health and ageing topic reviews both made recommendations bearing on the research framework. The mental health review notes that 'The study of whole systems emerged as a priority', even though the majority of suggestions 'were general statements about different services' (Department of Health, 1999f, p.16). The report on ageing makes the point even more strongly:

> The ultimate systems model for evaluation of health services is the
> population laboratory in which an epidemiological study identifies all
> people in a defined population who have a particular problem and
> then traces them through the health care system with or without
> embedded randomised trials. ... This form of study is expensive
> and only feasible where funding from more than one agency is

available. It is therefore difficult to replicate and in many instances comparison of several subsystems may be a more cost-effective use of research funds.

Department of Health, 1999c, p.17

The complexity of health care is only just being recognised as its central feature (Plsek and Greenhalgh, 2001). The main consequence, as far as research is concerned, is that it is risky to focus on one area in isolation from others. Yet that is the central methodological technique across virtually all clinical research and much health services research.

The need to think in systems terms either at the level of large patient groups such as those identified in the national service frameworks, or functions such as the provision of emergency care, may seem obvious. Yet to do so not only cuts across the existing research tradition, but also has to overcome strong forces pushing in the other direction, in particular the growth of specialisation driven in large measure by the products of the health research economy.

The spread of specialisation poses fundamental problems in the health research economy: what the structure should be for thinking about research requirements, what groups of disciplines and institutional forms are appropriate and how the work of different disciplines should be combined (Gelijns *et al.*, 1998).[51] As we have argued elsewhere (Harrison, 2001), it is not self-evident how national health care systems should be deconstructed into subsidiary systems – whether by client group, disease or care process – and how the sub-systems should relate to each other. Essentially the same issue arises in thinking about what the structure should be for the provider of the research economy.

As emphasised by the King's Fund evidence cited in the previous chapter, and the topic review of ageing and the Foresight report, the NHS is faced with a series of interlocking issues regarding the design of service delivery which require a scale of response which no existing institution could put together.

---

51. This not just a problem for the public sector. Gelijns and colleagues argue: 'The central issue is how to establish institutional arrangements that promote dialogue and cooperation among academic disciplines and departments, especially in the face of possible organisational disincentives. Even in industry, in which product-related research and development is highly interdisciplinary, development teams should resist the temptation to focus narrowly on expected indications' (Gelijns *et al.*, 1998, p.695).

The Foresight 2020 report, for example, proposed that:

> *a health care 'laboratory' is established to model the impact on demand for care of technological, demographic and other trends. ... This should not be in a single site but based on a flexible multi-site collaboration.*

> DTI/OST 2001, p.11

Whether it will prove possible to put together research groupings covering the range of disciplines envisaged in the Foresight report is far from clear. There are no organisations which have the capacity to synthesise knowledge from such a wide range of disciplines and which also have the capacity to turn such a synthesis into implementable plans for change. In principle universities may do this, but they are subject to pressures which push in the other direction, i.e. in favour of excellence within traditional disciplinary boundaries.

Policy response

Strengthening capacity

Despite the series of reports and initiatives cited above, the consultation paper on NHS Priorities and Needs Funding accepted that capacity was still deficient:

> *5.1 The right research capacity is required to give the NHS timely access to high quality evidence. There are research skill shortages in a range of health sectors such as public health and primary care, in some health professions and in several academic disciplines such as health economics. These limit the scope for R&D to generate the knowledge the NHS needs. NHS Priorities and Needs Funding will contribute to work to develop this capacity.*

It goes on to indicate that:

> *5.2 It will develop research capacity for the NHS by promoting:*

> ■ *an environment which supports and values the development of research skills and experience*
> ■ *access to research training opportunities*

■ *access to resources to undertake research activity*
■ *secure and attractive pathways for researchers and research-active practitioners.*

The Department of Health and the NHS will identify where skill shortages are most damaging and urgent. In the context of its strategic alliance with the HEFCE and concordats with the research councils, the Department will harmonise its approach to capacity planning with the HEFCE and our research funding partners.

Department of Health, 2000e, p.15

The Department of Health's paper on R&D within public health also indicated that action was being taken to address the supply side:

A research capacity strategy group is undertaking a programme of work which includes:

■ *quantifying the present stock of academic posts in order to better inform a strategy for building academic capacity, and in particular, to enable identified areas of shortage to be addressed*
■ *establishing new research training opportunities ... to develop a cadre of research leaders for the immediate and medium term future ... including ...*
  – 'career scientist' awards ...
  – 'Health of the Public' fellowships ...

funding for the awards has been made available from the Public Health Development Fund, DH, and the MRC. Discussions are taking place with relevant bodies, particularly universities, about longer term support for these initiatives.

Department of Health, 2001c, p.23

In 2000, a workforce capacity development project was established. The project was to be managed by a Workforce Capacity Implementation Group (now called the Research and Development Workforce Capacity Strategy Group). This was set up to investigate: 'issues relating to capacity building across all NHS disciplines and healthcare settings' (Department of Health, 2002c).

The group established a series of subgroups looking at specific disciplines poorly represented in the research field, including those discussed above. It also set in train a number of other projects, some aimed at establishing the current situation, e.g. a stocktake of R&D skills in public health, and established new awards for public health scientists and primary care.[52] In March 2001 the National Clinical Scientists scheme was launched 'to address longstanding concerned about clinical academic careers', following publication in March 2001 of a report from the Academy of Medical Science (Savill, 2000).

However, the position statement issued in February 2001 acknowledged that 'there are research skill shortages in health sectors including public health and primary care, some health professions, and several academic disciplines. These limit the scope for NHS R&D to generate the knowledge the NHS needs' (Department of Health, 2001f, para.6.1). It indicates that there will be a national budget to develop and maintain this capacity and outlines a series of other measures designed to support the supply of research including research focused on areas discussed above, such as nursing, primary care and public health.

Broad or narrow focus

In many areas of research, teams based on a single discipline or field may be the prerequisite for developing expertise. In the case of nursing, for example, the Department of Health's paper *Towards a Strategy for Nursing Research and Development* argues:

> that the Department [should] explore options for pump-priming a handful of designated centres with thematic research and development programmes to help build capacity through partnerships and collaboration focusing on links with the NHS and service delivery.

> Department of Health, 2000a, p.6

The report goes on to make further institutional proposals (see the box overleaf) designed to overcome the insularity of existing professional structures. The same approach was adopted in the early 1990s for primary care with the establishment of the National Centre.

In other areas of research, as noted in the 'Organisations' section above, there are pressures for a more collaborative, interdisciplinary approach.

---

52. Fuller details are available at the Department of Health website.

TOWARDS A STRATEGY FOR NURSING RESEARCH AND DEVELOPMENT

22. There is a strong case for additional investment to seed and develop a handful of designed centres of expertise. These centres should have well established research capacity and infrastructure. Each would be required to focus on an NHS priority and to work (through a hub and spoke system) with less developed units to engage, advise and support and link to programmes and projects, and to build research training circuits with pre and post-doctoral opportunities. A good model is the MRC Health Service Research collaboration. A relatively small additional investment could yield a substantial return on investment because of the way in which established centres are able to pool income streams to make in-house expertise available across programmes and projects.

23. Majoring on one of the NHS priorities such as cancer, mental health or CHD, each designed centre would focus on a thematic programme of R&D activity. The hub or centre (which could be virtual) would include expertise in, for example, economics, statistics and psychology in addition to nursing. This hub would link with less developed units (spokes), each linked with service providers in primary, secondary and tertiary care. The centres would serve as a locus for high quality research and development, training and supervision, and hence for generating capacity. There would be clear career plans with opportunities for joint clinical and research careers. The centres could be pump primed by the NHS Research and Development programme, possibly in conjunction with the Higher Education Funding Council, research councils and charities, and then be expected to generate, within 5–10 years, their own external grant income to sustain the programme of capacity building.

(Department of Health, 2000a, p.5)

This need for collaboration between research groups defined by disciplines or specific fields has in part been recognised. The Department of Health proposes:

> to improve the coherence between research activity that is devolved to the NHS and its academic partners on the one hand, and centrally managed R&D programmes on the other. The aim is to place much R&D of national priority with NHS/academic research groupings that

have the right expertise, experience and strategic R&D management capacity. These groupings would be collaborations of NHS organisations, academic units and, where appropriate, other partners, often working across local health communities or systems, or within specific networks of services or care pathways.

Department of Health, 2000f, p.12[53]

We have yet to see what this means in practice.

Overview

A number of general themes emerge from the examples considered in the first part of this chapter:

- There are cultural obstacles to research within the non-medical professions.
- Many areas lack a research base in organisational terms.
- Links between researchers working on the same topic are often poor.
- The current funding structure does not encourage the development of research capacity in new areas.

Taken together these represent substantial barriers to the development of significant research programmes in areas where the provider base is weak. Furthermore, the weakness of the provider side has been recognised for over a decade, suggesting that the obstacles to improvement are very substantial.

While changes to funding structures may help, it is clear they are not enough in themselves. The range of actions identified in successive reports indicate that, if the concentration on medical research identified in 1988 is to be remedied, a sustained and broad-based policy effort will be required.

The measures the Department of Health has undertaken are clearly moving in the right direction, but they remain modest in scope. Even if they are successful, it will be some time before the supply side of the

---

53. The government response to the Roberts (2002) report in its 2002 comprehensive spending review suggests that the difficulties faced by the health research economy have been recognised as part of a more general problem in publicly funded research.

health research economy is able to respond to new demands
upon it. As things stand, therefore, it is clear that difficulties with the
supply of the necessary research skills are an effective constraint on how
fast the programme can be rebalanced into new or less well-established
fields.

While the obstacles facing individual researchers, professions and topic
areas are of course important, a more fundamental issue is whether the
institutions currently in place are of the right type. Clearly some narrowly
focused research teams are fit for purpose and the establishment of new
centres may be appropriate for areas where the main need is to develop
a research tradition. In other areas, such an approach may not be
appropriate. It remains to be seen, however, whether collaborative
approaches across a wide range of disciplines are feasible, what practical
steps the Department of Health proposes to bring them about and
whether those steps will prove effective.

Institutional change alone is unlikely to be enough. Other supply side
constraints must be removed, particularly those associated with
professions and disciplines. Some actual and proposed changes
elsewhere are hopeful. For some time now there have been experiments
with interdisciplinary learning. The report of the Bristol Inquiry (Kennedy,
2001) argued strongly for this, in the light of its analysis of poor
communication between professionals as being one of the main
sources of failure. Though addressed to hospitals, it applies equally
to the effective working of the supply side of the research economy.
As developments such as this feed through into the workforce, some of
the difficulties identified here will become soluble. But they will have
little impact unless the demand side of the research economy changes
in step with it.

Chapter 6

Inter-relationships and co-ordination

There are important connections between all the players in the health research economy. This chapter looks at initiatives to co-ordinate the research effort within the public sector and at the relatively limited attempts to define the role of the public sector in the light of the contribution of the private for-profit and not-for-profit sectors.

6 Inter-relationships and co-ordination

Chapters 1 and 2 showed that the health research economy is diverse, with different parts of it subject to different incentives and disincentives. Furthermore, although each of the providers and funders is to some extent self-contained, there are important connections between them.

These interconnections are of various sorts:

- There are potential overlaps in research funding, i.e. more than one funder may support the same line of research. This means that, to avoid wasteful overlap, the various players should achieve sensible division of roles on a pragmatic basis.
- Different elements need to co-operate either to carry out research or to provide the basis for it, for example in large-scale clinical trials, but the incentives they are subject to may make co-operation unattractive.
- Research may require access to facilities used by non-research activities, e.g. the patients and treatment facilities of the hospital. The research hospital is a point of intersection between service delivery, teaching and research, with potential conflicts between them.

The first part of this chapter considers the quest for co-ordination within the public sector. Here the issue is partly one of avoiding overlap and partly one of ensuring that independent agencies within the public part of the health research economy align their behaviour with the 'needs of the NHS' and health policy in general.

We then take the private sector into account. As pointed out in Chapter 2, there are areas of research which the private sector may be unwilling to carry out. Such gaps are in part filled by public agencies. Another approach is to modify the framework within which the private sector operates. This may involve the introduction of new players or other targeted measures designed to bring private incentives and public needs into line. It is here that the Department of Health has a key role. The Department does not and cannot plan the health research economy and its role as a payer is relatively modest. But it can adapt its own role and attempt to modify the roles of others. We look at these issues in the second part of this chapter.

The search for a 'co-ordinated' system

The 1988 House of Lords report

The 1988 report again provides our starting point. While it accepted that the health research economy should be diverse, it found that there was no co-ordination between the public sector payers and providers.

In its response, the Government attempted to find a compromise between allowing 'competitive' forces to prevail and avoiding wasteful duplication:

> *2.17 Together with the Select Committee, the Government wishes to retain and foster this diversity which is a source of strength. It rejects pressures for central control and monopoly. Steps will be taken to enhance exchanges of information between the bodies concerned, which with cross-membership of committees will help duplication to be avoided and gaps to be filled. The Government believes that co-ordination on individual issues is best met by mechanisms designed to meet specific needs, rather than an over-arching and perhaps over-bureaucratic committee. Decisions on priorities in research should be left to individual agencies – over most of which the Government rightly has little or no direct control and does not intend to seek it.*

> Department of Health, 1989, p.6

Not surprisingly, given the nature of the then Government, it preferred to co-ordinate the various interests represented in the health research economy through the provision of information about the kinds of work which should be supported in the expectation that the actors would respond by modifying or developing their contribution. It therefore went on to indicate that the new Director of R&D would 'have an important role in representing the interest of the Department of Health and the NHS in the wider research community' (Department of Health, 1989, para.2.20). 'Representing' implies at best influence, and certainly not control.

In 1993 *Research for Health* set out a similar approach when it acknowledged the need for effective links between the various members of the pluralist research system and set out a number of measures to achieve this. In particular it noted that:

> To promote better understanding of respective strategies and priorities, a number of research liaison committees (RLCs) have been convened to bring together public and private research funding bodies. ... The purpose is to identify gaps in the overall coverage of research, to be aware of potentially unproductive duplication and to examine the advantages of complementary strategies and opportunities for collaboration on specific projects.

Department of Health, 1993, p.5

Concordats and other bilateral arrangements

There followed a number of bilateral initiatives between the main players, supported by a large number of committees and other formal structures designed to co-ordinate their activities. We have already noted the concordat reached between the Department of Health and the MRC as a successor to the ill-fated Rothschild arrangements. That was renewed in 1992[54] and was designed to:

- ensure co-ordination in their missions and strategic planning and that their research activities complement one another
- ensure that health department policies and priorities are informed by scientific advances and opportunities and that health department research needs are understood and addressed by the MRC
- ensure that the NHS and public health perspectives are understood and taken account of by the MRC in decisions on research funding and to ensure that the needs of the MRC research for NHS support are understood and addressed.

(adapted from Department of Health, 1998c)

The concordat rests on a broad division of roles, but one which cannot not be clear-cut. It states that:

> Whereas basic medical research (whether biological or clinical) is the responsibility of the MRC, there are overlapping responsibilities of the MRC and Health departments in applied research, including health

---

54. The MRC website (mrc.ac.uk) contains the 1997 version of the concordat. The broad aims remain unchanged.

services research and applied clinical research. Operational research and health related surveillance will generally be the responsibility of the Health departments who also have an interest in research which may be outside the MRC's prime sphere of interest including, for example, aspects of economics, social science and engineering.

MRC, 1992, para.4

The *de facto* dividing line between the Department and the MRC can only be determined pragmatically through sharing of information and other informal means of co-ordination.

In 1994 the MRC published *Priorities for Health: The research response* in which it set out what it was doing of direct relevance to the Department of Health. In subsequent years, the MRC published a number of research and topic overviews relevant to the NHS and the Department of Health. The MRC acknowledges that its priorities have been modified in the light of priorities within the Department of Health. For example, a report issued in 1994 notes that:

The change of culture and organisation within the NHS has demanded the definition of a new research agenda.

MRC, 1994a, p.3

In addition, the MRC has set out in a number of papers its views on broad sectors and also set out its own priorities. These enable other elements of the research economy to form their own judgement about how their contributions might relate to what the MRC is supporting.

A similar concordat was reached with the Economic and Social Research Council (ESRC) in 1983. This notes that the two partners in the concordat have a shared interest in:

■ *management, organisation and cost effectiveness of health and social services, measurement and evaluation of health status, outcomes in the health and personal social services, and quality of life*
■ *evaluation of community care policy*
■ *social, geographical and economic variations in health and well being*
■ *health-related behaviours and lifestyles*
■ *evaluation of health and social care policies.*

It then states that:

5. *The ESRC and DoH will consider addressing these areas of shared interest in one or more of the following ways:*
   a. *input to scientific reviews, workshops and consultations to identify research or training priorities*
   b. *consultation regarding peer review of research proposals and results*
   c. *joint or co-funding of research, research resources or training*
   d. *ESRC management of DoH funded initiatives in areas of mutual interest*
   e. *exploration of scope for closer co-operation on international research into health and social services*
   f. *exploration of areas of common interest in review and dissemination of information from R&D programmes*
   g. *co-operation on training and career development of social scientists in health and social services research and in health economics*
   h. *developing liaison between social scientists and NHS regional research and, where appropriate, helping social scientists form collaborative contacts with the regions, and other health and social care agencies.*

   Unpublished mimeo

Concordats have also been reached with the other research councils.[55]

A similar arrangement was agreed between the Department of Health and the HEFCE (Department of Health/HEFCE, 2000) The overall purpose of this was described as follows:

2. *The Statement of Alliance builds upon existing arrangements of good liaison, formal consultation, and representation on key advisory and decision-making bodies. It provides the foundation and the framework for the DH and HEFCE to take strategic and longer-term views on issues of shared interest, and to develop plans which may transcend institutional, disciplinary and professional boundaries.*

---

55. The Department of Health website refers to these and provides a hyperlink to the Natural Environment Research Council with which a concordat was reached in 2001. This, like the other concordats, embodies agreements to exchange information and work together in areas of mutual interest.

3. *Working together through a new Strategic Alliance, the DH and the HEFCE will support policies, initiatives and programmes which deliver public policy objectives for health and social care research. This research will have impacts on the health and social services and on policy making.*

Department of Health/HEFCE, 2000

It goes on to note that the responsibilities of the two parties:

5. *HEFCE has responsibility for funding infrastructure in higher education institutions (HEIs). HEFCE's criteria for allocating infrastructure funds will need to take proper account of the needs of those in the health and social care research fields for relevant and applicable research.*
6. *DH has responsibility for funding the research infrastructure within the NHS, which will need to be integrated with HEFCE-supported provision in associated HEIs. Normally this will mean integration at the local level. On occasion it will also require integration across geographical areas to ensure the necessary infrastructure is in place and the workforce has the necessary research capacity and capability.*

Department of Health/HEFCE, 2000

These general statements in themselves are hard to fault, but their very lack of specificity means that neither side is committed to particular activities. However, the process of defining the Alliance led to the identification of nursing and allied health professions as the area most in need of action to develop research capacity: the reports noted in Chapter 5 have been the initial result (HEFCE/JM Consulting, 20002a and b).

The National Forum

Over and above such bilateral agreements, a National Forum was established to further exchange between all the main players in the health research economy. Its original terms of reference are in the box opposite.

The National Forum consists of representatives from the health departments, the NHS and the other main funding agencies in the public and private sector. Its proceedings are not in the public domain.

NATIONAL FORUM TERMS OF REFERENCE

1. The National Forum provides a forum for funders of medical and health services research to meet and consider issues of mutual interest, in relation to R&D in, and relevant to, health.

2. The National Forum will share information and exchange views on:

    i.   current national and international strategic issues relating to research and health services research and development and other issues of R&D that are of importance to the health

    ii. the overall pattern of funding for research and development in medical and health services research

    iii. the plans, priorities and funding arrangements of individual medical and health services research funding agencies, in particular new systems of funding and supporting research and development in the NHS

    iv. the development of systems for information about medical and health services research activity

    v.   the development of research capacity in medical and health service research, particularly that needed by the NHS

    vi. advances in science and technology which may impact on health care

    vii. technology transfer, covering links between basic science, applied research and health services.

(Department of Health, 1995f – the new Terms of Reference are described rather more succinctly on the Department of Health website)

Cross-agency working on specific topics

In addition to these overarching relationships, a considerable number of other structures, e.g. liaison committees, have developed, focusing on particular research areas such as cardiovascular disease and biomedical technology (see House of Lords, 1995, p.11).

These are precisely the kind of arrangement that public sector bureaucracies use to 'co-ordinate' their work, i.e. a massive array of interlocking committees. From the outside there is no way of knowing how well or how badly they operate.

There are instances where they appear to work well. For example, the DTI's LINK research programme appears to be working effectively across the public/private sector boundary. The Department of Health has also participated in the Teaching Company Scheme (which promotes technology transfer between academic institutions and industry), sponsoring work in the area of rehabilitation devices. In March 2000 the Department of Trade and Industry, the Wellcome Trust and the HEFCE announced a joint scheme to fund research into heart disease and the workings of the human brain (DTI, 2000a).

Examples such as Foresight and the ESRC programme on Innovative Health Technologies[56] can also be found where projects have been generated which represent explicit attempts to work across conventional subject and organisational boundaries.

But, drawing again from recent policy papers, we can infer that the Department of Health has accepted that the existing co-ordination mechanisms can be improved. *Research and Development for a First Class Service* indicates the Department's intention to:

■ work with the main R&D funding bodies in 2000 to define initial standards of strategic direction, mutual influence, open access and quality assurance
■ develop joint mechanisms to discuss strategic direction, priorities, standards and processes at the working level
■ clarify the contribution of other R&D funders to supporting clinical, public health and health services R&D
■ build on the already close partnership set out in the Concordats with the research councils, to refine information sharing and joint planning
■ develop the Statement of Partnership with other research funding bodies into an agreement based on clear standards and mutual obligations and
■ enter into a formal Strategic Alliance with HEFCE.
(Department of Health, 2000b)

The same point is noted in *A Research and Development Strategy for Public Health*. The paper argues that:

lack of co-ordination across funding agencies leads to lost potential for complete understanding of particular public health issues, for

---

56. The central question this addresses is: How will people and society be affected by, and in turn affect, innovative health technologies?

*identifying and addressing gaps in the evidence base, for promoting
multi-disciplinary research, and for encouraging widespread
dissemination and use of research results.*

Department of Health, 2001c, p.7

As the paper makes clear, the public health research economy is more
complex than that for health services. A much larger array of public
agencies is involved. Many of these, for example those responsible for
agriculture, transport and the environment, do not see themselves as
being involved in public health research. Bureaucratic exchange through
committees may be insufficient to engage them fully, since each has its
own priorities and calls on research funds. The topic review on accidents
no doubt reflects such differences. It states that:

*In Britain, ownership of the injury problem, its solutions and research
is fragmented ... This review has highlighted the need for collaborative
research across all types of accidental injury from causation right
through to rehabilitation of the injured.*

Department of Health, 1999h, p.76

But there are no obvious solutions to the obstacles posed by the
boundaries between areas of responsibility. In other areas the present
Government has introduced measures designed to weld together the
activities of various parts of Government, one example being the
Deprivation Unit in the Cabinet Office. These measures have addressed
issues of particular political salience and where action has enjoyed the
Prime Minister's support. The public health agenda has not enjoyed that
degree of political exposure, despite successive green and white papers
(Department of Health, 1999b) to which many departments have
contributed. The same is true of action to tackle particular diseases which
would involve a wide range of organisations (some of them not primarily
health organisations), were a comprehensive approach to be
implemented.

The interface between the universities and the NHS

Mechanisms for cross-boundary working

Within the health sector itself there are important interfaces between the
universities and the NHS itself: both have a role in the training of
clinicians and the teaching and research hospital has been a central

feature of the health research economy since the early part of the 20th century. These interfaces have proved very troublesome from the viewpoint not only of research, but also of teaching and care. They, too, have given rise to a large number of committees and reports.

In 1990 the Standing Group on University Medical and Dental Education and Research (SGUMDER) set out ten principles which should govern relationships between medical schools and teaching hospitals (see box opposite). Though bearing primarily on training, the principles have implications for research as well.

These principles, slightly modified since their original formulation, have been endorsed by the Secretaries of State for Health, for Education and Science and for Scotland and have been promulgated to the NHS and to the universities.

This SGUMDER report was one of several appearing during the 1990s designed to get relationships between the universities and the health sector right, including further reports from SGUMDER, the higher education funding councils, the Joint Medical Advisory Committee and the Department of Health. In 1997, the Department of Health commissioned two task groups to help develop relationships between the NHS and academic institutions (see Smith, 2001, for a summary of each report).

These were followed up in 1999 with *Good Practice in NHS/Academic Links*, commissioned by the Joint Medical Advisory Committee (HEFCE, 1999). The report aimed to 'identify issues relating to the interface between the NHS and universities, to highlight places where these issues are being dealt with effectively and to promote good practice'.

These documents represent a substantial response to the interface issue. They are too detailed to go into here, but their very existence can be taken as evidence that the various interfaces have not been working well and that further efforts are required to help them to do so. Two recent publications from the Nuffield Trust focusing on the interface between the NHS and universities confirm this (Nuffield Trust, 2000; Smith, 2001). Both suggest that the pressures in different parts of the health research economy and the context in which it operates have worked against their effective collaborative working, despite the efforts to move them together. The HEFCE report, however, does cite a number of 'good practices' where it appears that effective working across organisation and activity boundaries has been achieved.

THE REVISED 'TEN KEY PRINCIPLES'

Strategic principles

1. The aim of the undergraduate medical and dental education is to produce doctors and dentists who are able to meet the present and future health and health care needs. To this end, future doctors and dentists should be educated in an atmosphere which combines high professional standards with a spirit of intellectual enquiry and innovation based on active research and development programmes.
2. The objective of medical and dental research is to maintain and improve the nation's health and health care by contributing to the promotion of health and the understanding of disease.
3. The universities and the NHS have a shared responsibility for ensuring high standards are achieved and maintained in undergraduate medical and dental education and in research.

Operational principles

4. The local provision of undergraduate medical and dental education, guided by clearly defined and co-ordinated national policies must be supported by effective joint planning at a local level.
5. Universities, health authorities, trusts and, where appropriate, GP fundholders, should share relevant information and consult one another about their plans. Once established, policies and plans should be disseminated locally and reviewed regularly.
6. The NHS and universities should consult one another about the special interest and contribution to service, teaching and research of senior medical and dental appointments.
7. Where agreement cannot be reached locally, the NHS Executive Regional Director and the Vice-Chancellor of the University should confer.

Funding principles

8. The NHS and universities should ensure that undergraduate medical and dental education and research are undertaken efficiently and cost-effectively.
9. The universities and NHS should work closely together in funding research and development within the NHS in England.
10. SIFT should be allocated on the basis of mutually agreed service plans to support teaching. Universities should be joint signatories to all SIFT contracts.

(Smith, 2001)

The central Nuffield criticism is that the issues are not addressed 'in the round', but on a piecemeal basis. The first paper found that:

> *Bodies that address NHS/university relations tend to focus on aspects of the problem. Issues around service provision, particularly, are less prominent in this agenda. There is a need for the parties who are operationally responsible for the successful management of the tripartite mission to take a strategic approach at UK level, to both guide and represent the development of local University Clinical Centres.*

Nuffield Trust, 2000, para.68

To address this situation, the paper concluded, requires:

> *a UK forum for Academic Clinical Partnership and for considering whether there is a need to rationalise other existing bodies at the national level that address the NHS/university interface.*

Nuffield Trust, 2000, para.69

A forum, however, would not be enough – the second report goes on to say that in addition:

> *There is a need to marry up the R&D [NHS] and RAE [university] research objectives. At the root of increased tensions in recent years are the conflicting objectives of research strategies. In the competition for research funds universities have adopted strategies that focus on their strengths, particularly basic science. There is a perception that the RAE has downgraded clinical research and a need to redefine it and increase its credibility. How this is seen in the next RAE will be defining, it will be an opportunity to align the two research agendas.*

Smith, 2001, para.87

Although this point is made in the context of medical schools and teaching hospitals, it is a general one running across the NHS/ Department of Health/university interface. The issue is one of conflicting incentives. Quality control methods promoted in the university sector do not encourage some of the kinds of work the NHS needs, rather the reverse. Part of the difficulty faced by professions such as nursing or pharmacy in developing research programmes within a university environment has been due to the criteria used in the research assessment exercise (RAE) to which the universities have been subject. These criteria did not reflect the need for at least some research to engage with the NHS.[57]

The same point is noted in *A Research and Development Strategy for Public Health* which indicates that the HEFCE:

> '*has noted the need to ensure that multi-disciplinary research is valued appropriately for the research assessment exercise and has made a number of important changes to the rules for the 2001 RAE exercise to reassure researchers that this form of research will be properly assessed.*

Department of Health, 2001c, para.6.11

Whether this will prove effective remains to be seen, but it is in any case only part of a larger problem. This assessment process reflects the persistent divide between what is highly valued within the academic part of the health research economy and that which the NHS needs. As a leader article in the *Pharmaceutical Journal* put it:

> *So, researchers with good work in the pharmacy practice areas will try to get their paper into a journal with a high impact factor, which, in practice, means publishing outside the profession. This means that that work will not be widely seen by practising pharmacists. The whole process is driven by academic aspirations rather than the needs of practice. There also seems to be a view – and this can be discerned from the task force's report – that publication in a health and social sciences journal is first rate, whereas publication in a pharmacy journal is second rate. Researchers need to align their loyalties.*

Pharmaceutical Journal, 1 February 1997, 258: 153

---

57. See *The Times Higher Education Supplement*, 21/28 December 2001, for a report on this issue in the latest RAE: 'It is really an invidious position. We have argued for not reducing the pretty small share of the pot that grade-3 departments get. This research has real potential. In other disciplines, such as health studies, a grade 4 could be received by people working on the ground with particular projects and it is important that the research is financed.'

A report from the Scottish Universities Research Policy Consortium (2002) acknowledges that 'certain type of niche research may sometimes exist in departments with a lower rating yet still be of immense value to its users'. However, it put the onus firmly on the universities to deal with the problem (section 4.2.10).

Those wanting to succeed in the academic field are encouraged to examine topics and use methodologies which lead to problems being ignored – problems which those providing services nevertheless have to tackle.

The incentive issue is part of a wider interface issue bearing on the full range of NHS/Department of Health/university relationships. These can quite appropriately be of various kinds, ranging from one-off contracting to the establishment of specialist centres. Looked at from the Department of Health/NHS angle, the key issue is whether the university sector can provide the right types of 'production facility', i.e. the right combination of skills and disciplines to meet its knowledge requirements. Taking a wider view, the question is whether the overall contribution of the university sector is appropriate, given the roles of the other players in the health research economy – in particular, whether the universities can continue with the role they are uniquely placed to carry out.

The implications of the university funding system

The main distinctive contribution of the sector is 'disinterested study and expertise' – a role which allows it to monitor the workings of the other elements independently of any of them and to choose its own areas of investigation. The system for financing the university sector, embodying as it does a degree of block finance, in principle provides the scope for this. But this role is to some extent under threat through the development of more effective links between the universities and other parts of the health research economy.

As far as links with the public sector are concerned, the issues have already been touched on in the previous chapter. The supply side of the health research economy within the university sector is not in general financially secure, with consequences for the careers of individuals in health-related research. Reliance on external sources to some degree limits the independence of the university sector and its ability to research into areas which funders are not interested in.

In addition, the university sector in general is being encouraged to 'act entrepreneurially', i.e. to develop businesses out of their own intellectual capital themselves or to enter into various forms of partnerships with the private sector. In 2001, for example, the Trade and Industry Secretary invited bids from the university sector for funds to turn bright ideas into commercial successes (DTI, 2001c). Announcing the scheme, he described the universities as 'engines of growth'.

Viewed from the standpoint of the Department of Trade and Industry, where they are successful, initiatives of this kind appear obviously beneficial. Looked at from the standpoint of the Department of Health they may bring costs as well as benefits – the potential loss of the disinterested source of expertise and the translation into private goods of what might formerly have been public property. This latter process may well encourage innovation, but may also discourage it by reducing the (relatively) free exchange which typifies the workings of the academic community.

The issues touched on here are very complex and we cannot tackle them in detail. The central question is whether there is an effective process which does or could tackle them: the answer appears to be no. The Nuffield papers bring out clearly the fact that a way has not been found within the NHS of considering simultaneously the various elements which must, as things currently stand, mesh together within teaching and research hospitals. As we suggested in the previous chapter, however, whether the kind of relationships which exist now are the right ones and whether there are alternatives which would reduce the strains between the different functions is open to question. But what is clear is that these issues have yet to receive systematic investigation by all the interested parties and that there is no clear arena for this to be done.

This point is as true of the wider picture as it is of medical schools/research trusts in particular. The 'privatisation' of knowledge by encouraging researchers to patent and market the results of their work may be effective in encouraging the development of some new products of benefit to the NHS. But if it is carried too far, such a process may in fact be inefficient, to the extent that it leads to duplication of work. This may come about because researchers have a strong incentive to be secretive about what they do[58] and also because the process reduces the effectiveness of the free interchange of knowledge that characterises the non-commercial part of the health research economy, nationally and internationally.

---

58. This point is often made about research carried out in and for the pharmaceutical industry.

Public and private roles

Partnerships across the public–private interface

Because the NHS has never attempted to be a drugs producer in its own right, the existing division of roles between public and private sectors appears a natural one. But the terms of this partnership, as it is now referred to, have never been clearly defined across the full range of issues which it involves.

It has been accepted, however, that one element of this partnership should be public support for fundamental or pure research. The House of Lords 1988 report argued that:

> *6.6 The Committee believes that it is reasonable for the industry to look to the Government to support the essential research base. The ABPI's evidence on this point was cogent*

> House of Lords, 1988, QQ 129, 156–8

This role is suited to Government because pure research is high risk and there are benefits from its results being public rather than private goods. What the scale and focus of this support should be are other matters, and neither has received any systematic attention in official papers. Implicitly the question is answered through the level of resources allocated to the MRC and arguably the HEFCE.

Nevertheless the private sector is dependent on the public sector in respect of basic research and the organisation of major trials, while the NHS has always largely relied on the private sector for the development of new drugs and medical devices. This complementary relationship has been to a great extent taken for granted since the foundation of the NHS. Recently it was endorsed in the NHS Plan which set out a number of proposals for making the partnership between public and private sectors work better:

> *11.13 Advances in science and technology have revolutionised modern medicine, providing the antibiotics, vaccines, modern anaesthetics and pharmaceuticals that have helped transform our lives. The NHS has a responsibility to contribute to, facilitate and embrace these advances in partnership with the private and charitable sectors and academia.*

11.15 Working with the private sector and other partners we will commission NHS research and development in new centres of excellence.

Department of Health, 2000j

For obvious enough reasons the links between the pharmaceutical industry and the Department of Health have been strong since the 1950s when the first voluntary agreement between industry and Department was reach over the price of drugs. The latest report on what became the Pharmaceutical Price Regulation Scheme (Department of Health, 2000d) indicates that the scheme is designed to:

- secure the provision of safe and effective medicines for the NHS at reasonable cost
- promote a strong and profitable pharmaceutical industry capable of such sustained research and development as should lead to the future availability of new and improved medicines
- encourage the efficient and competitive development and supply of medicines to pharmaceutical markets in the UK and other countries.

Thus the agreement, which remains voluntary and non-statutory, is designed to strike a balance between the interests of the NHS and those of the companies supplying it. A key part of that balance is the perceived need to support a key part of the UK's science base and one of its most successful industrial sectors.

This theme was developed further with the establishment of the Pharmaceutical Industry Competitiveness Task Force in March 2000. This was set up to:

bring together the expertise and experience of the industry leaders in the UK with Government policy makers to identify and report to the Prime Minister on the steps that may need to be taken to retain and strengthen the competitiveness of the UK business environment for the innovative pharmaceutical industry.

Department of Health, 2001a

The Task Force focused on six areas:

- developments in the UK market
- intellectual property rights

- the regulation of medicines licensing
- the science base and biopharmaceuticals
- clinical research
- the wider economic climate.

As the items in the list show, the private sector 'needs' the public. Chapter 2 noted the importance of the legal and regulatory framework and also the support for basic research which the private sector is unlikely to fund itself. As for clinical research, if the private sector is to be able to develop products effectively through clinical trials, it requires close links with the NHS in its role of care provider.

The Task Force identifies five areas where improvements are required:

1. *Work by industry, the Department of Health (DH) and the NHS significantly to improve start up times on clinical trials from April 2001.*
2. *Development of a Research Governance Framework by DH which defines quality standards and clarifies responsibilities for all research involving patients in the NHS.*
3. *Development of a partnership agreement which defines the working relationship between industry and the NHS.*
4. *Work to improve transparency in costing and hence reduce transaction costs for commercial clinical trials.*
5. *Agreement of performance indicators to monitor progress and ongoing competitiveness of the UK in industry sponsored clinical research.*

Department of Health, 2001a

Evidence received by the Science and Technology Committee review of cancer research suggested that there was no clarity on the terms of this partnership in respect of items 4 and 5 (House of Commons, 2000). It revealed that there was no consistency in charging for the use of hospital facilities across the NHS. Whereas the Royal Pharmaceutical Society of Great Britain, speaking on behalf of hospital pharmacists, suggested that charges were too low, the industry claimed that the UK was making itself uncompetitive by charging too much relative to other countries.[59] The Government response to the Committee's report did not deal with these

---

59. Recent reports on the relationship between higher education institutions and the charitable sector suggest that similar issues arise here: see HEFCE/JM Consulting (2002a and 2000b).

issues in any substantive way. The issue was, however, taken up by the Task Force which found:

> *6.15 Surveys across many companies suggest that between 1993 and 1998, the costs of Phase II–III clinical research in the UK increased by 50%. Compared with our close European partners, the UK is more expensive and the gap appears to be widening.*

Not surprisingly therefore the report goes on:

> *6.29 The Department of Health will review its guidance on the relationship between prices charged by the NHS and the cost of studies with the intention of improving the transparency and consistency of pricing. The review will be informed by evidence of variations in NHS approaches to pricing and the cost of industry of conducting its research in other major markets. The overall aim will be, within the constraints of EC law and Government policy for public services, to minimise impediments to the UK's competitiveness for clinical trials when compared with major EU and North American markets. This review will be completed by 30/06/01.*
>
> Department of Health, 2001a, p.62

The Task Force report also indicates that the informal partnership which underlies existing relationships is to be formalised:

> *6.31 A Research Partnership Agreement is to be drawn up between the UK pharmaceutical industry represented by the ABPI and the Department of Health/NHS, that acts as a framework for continued interaction. It will parallel that for non-commercial (charity) funded research (this to cover issues of mutual interest and arrangements for collaborative work, funding, timeliness, communication between companies and NHS bodies and the quality of research in the wider public interest). Following the development of a Research Partnership Agreement, Industry and Government will establish a formal mechanism to continue discussion.*
>
> Department of Health, 2001a, p.62

At the time of writing, part of the terms of this partnership had just been published (Department of Health, 2002b). The aim is to enable joint funding of trials which are important both to industry and the NHS and it provides for industry to contribute to the costs of the research infrastructure. The logic of joint funding of trials is explicitly based on the acknowledgement that there are areas where research is needed into medicines, but which the private sector is likely to ignore.

Other partnership arrangements have already been developed. In its paper *Science and Innovation Strategy* (Department of Health, 2001m), the Department of Health refers to the Medlink programme and the work of the Medical Devices Agency. Medlink was established in 1995 'to improve quality of life and the competitiveness of the UK medical systems industry by encouraging the development and uptake of advanced technologies through collaborative research in areas of clinical priority'. The immediate stimulus to its establishment was a report from the Advisory Council on Science and Technology (DTI/OST, 1993) which recommended the creation of a programme to support the exploitation of research allied to medical and health care. The Medlink programme has been running ever since, supporting such projects as the development of a new form of heart valve or improved walking frames.

In respect of the Medical Devices Agency, the *Science and Innovation Strategy* states that:

> *2.13 Within the UK, the MDA undertakes extensive dialogue with ABPI and with manufacturers during the development of new devices, provides test facilities for manufacturers developing wheelchairs and artificial limbs and it is running an increasing number of conferences with the industry as well as regular liaison meetings. The Department also advises the Engineering and Physical Sciences Research Council (EPSRC) on the running of the Integrated Healthcare Technologies (IntHeTech) sector within the Council's Innovative Manufacturing Initiative. IntHeTech aims to identify and resolve barriers to innovation in healthcare, and to identify new ways of working that have been successfully used in other manufacturing industries and could be applied within the healthcare industry to improve competitiveness.*

> Department of Health, 2001m

In September 2001, the Government announced new proposals for public–private co-operation:

> *Project proposals will be assessed by an expert group drawn from industry, universities and NHS. Key criteria for approval of projects will be innovation, scientific quality, clinical or healthcare need*

and commitment of the industrial partner to manufacture the final product.

Department of Health, 2001b

Thus, in line with its general policy towards the private sector, the Government is taking or is about to take a number of steps towards improving the private–public interface. These, however, are largely designed to support the role of the private rather than the public sector.

Identifying gaps left by 'market failure'

As we have seen already, the central criticism made in the 1988 House of Lords report was that the NHS was poor at articulating its own research requirements. We have also seen that there are areas of research which the private sector may, under the incentives currently obtaining, be reluctant to take on.

However, neither the NHS Plan nor the Pharmaceutical Industry Competitiveness Task Force considered which areas of research into drugs and devices might be desirable from the viewpoint of the NHS and its users but unattractive for the private sector to work in. With rare exceptions, official papers describing the publicly financed programme do not ask what the proper role of the public sector is, given the massive spending in the private pharmaceutical sector and the quite different scale of activity and market structure in the devices sector. Nor do the Foresight papers do this.

The issue arose very clearly in the House of Lords inquiry into complementary medicine (House of Lords, 2001a). The inquiry noted that spending within the R&D programme on complementary medicines was very limited. It was also limited within the 'industry' supplying such medicines and treatments. In sharp contrast to the pharmaceutical industry, much of this industry is small-scale and many of the products are not patentable. The Committee recommended:

that companies producing products used in CAM should invest more heavily in research and development.

House of Lords, 2001a, para.7.81

But there were strong reasons for thinking it unlikely that the companies would in fact do so. The Committee noted that there was no patent protection for most products in this area. Furthermore the research capacity does not exist and, as a result, there are few high-quality research proposals:

> *Despite a general perception that funding bodies are biased against their field, funding is available for good-quality applications in the UK. Both the Wellcome Trust and the Medical Research Council will fund CAM proposals if the science is of a high enough standard. The success rate for CAM applications to the Trust is actually higher than for 'conventional' research proposals. Nevertheless, the number of applications received is very small.*
>
> *Wellcome News, 2000*

The House of Lords Committee therefore made recommendations designed to create research capacity within the public arena without specifying the terms on which its results might be available to the commercial sector.

> *34. We recommend that universities and other higher education institutions provide the basis for a more robust research infrastructure in which CAM and conventional research and practice can take place side-by-side and can benefit from interaction and greater mutual understanding. We recommend that a small number of such centres of excellence, in or linked to medical schools, be established with the support of research funding agencies including the Research Councils, the Department of Health, Higher Education Funding Councils and the charitable sector.*
>
> House of Lords, 2001a, para.7.57[60]

The same issue arises with so-called orphan drugs, i.e. drugs which serve a market too small for the private sector to consider investing in it.[61] In late 2001, the Department of Health announced a modest programme of research in this area. The Medicines Control Agency (responsible for product licensing) encourages what it terms 'limited use' drugs by requiring less stringent safety and efficacy data, lower fees for approval

---

60. Similar recommendations are to be found in White House (2002).

61. The US Orphan Drug Act defines a rare disease as one which affects fewer than 200,000 people in the USA and for which no reasonable expectation exists that the costs of developing and distributing drugs to treat such disease will be recovered from the sales of the drugs.

and possible fast-track approval. A further policy response is in the process of being developed in the form of a European Directive which offers enhanced patent protection (Department of Health, 2000k).

However, that may not be enough. At the moment there is no clear locus for determining where such gaps might lie. When undertaking a strategic review of any disease or client group, the Department of Health/NHS should ask what the private sector is likely to supply or seek to supply, what topics it is likely to ignore and, of these, which may be worth exploring.

Dinsmore (2001), for example, makes the point that most research on the links between genes and health has been funded by the private sector, but the focus of this work has been drugs not on other links that might be more effective in promoting health, e.g. links bearing on the responsiveness of individuals to different forms of nutrition.

Another example is the potential value of drugs in areas for which they were not originally developed. Here there may be obstacles within both public and private sectors. According to Gelijns and colleagues:

> *The central issue is how to establish institutional arrangements that promote dialogue and cooperation among academic disciplines and departments, especially in the face of possible organizational disincentives. Even in industry, in which product-related research and development is highly interdisciplinary, development teams should resist the temptation to focus narrowly on expected indications.*

Gelijns *et al.*, 1998, p.695

They go on to argue that there is a need to provide additional private-sector incentives for research into 'secondary' uses of drugs:

> *Finally, clinical evaluative research is necessary to substantiate the new indications. If the expected market value is low, the public sector may be the only source of support. For example, the National Institutes of Health had to support the trials that evaluated the use of aspirin to prevent myocardial infarction, because pharmaceutical companies were not prepared to do so in light of the difficulty of obtaining exclusive economic benefits from the trials. Public-sector support for this type of research has, unfortunately, been limited. According to a recent report by the Panel on Clinical Research of the National*

Institutes of Health, only 27 per cent of all research funds awarded in fiscal year 1996 were partly or completely earmarked for clinical research, a category that includes but is not limited to clinical evaluative research.

Gelijns *et al.*, 1998, p.697

As the above example shows, there is a gap – in this case identified in the USA – which arises 'near the patient' after drugs have been identified and licensed where the private sector generally loses interest. The box below illustrates a similar kind of failure, this time arising in the case of surgery.

Yet another gap is caused by the tendency of innovative research to focus on the positive – the scope for therapeutic or other benefits – to the neglect of the possibly negative side effects. Yet governments persistently find themselves in the position of saying there is no evidence of harm (e.g. BSE transmission to humans) when no one has actually looked for such evidence.

To fill gaps of these kinds requires a more active public role than currently exists.

DISINCENTIVES TO SURGICAL RESEARCH

A further disincentive to doing surgical research, particularly surgery that involves a high capital cost for an implantable device, has been the reluctance of device manufacturers to take a role in funding the capital cost for these new pieces of surgical equipment. If a company is going to benefit from a higher share price, they should have, within the 'D' part of their R&D budget, some way of paying for the capital costs of their device whilst it is being evaluated. Within the pharmaceutical industry this is easier, in that the individual cost of the trial drug is small compared with the total investment, but this may not be the case for complex medical devices. Companies want rapid regulatory approval so that they can quickly go to the market. Not infrequently, a good trial is designed and set up but ultimately fails because the equipment is given marketing approval and then the company no longer wants to fund the trial.

(Johnston and Sussex, 2000, p.39)

Acting as an informed purchaser

To define this role involves being an informed purchaser or market manager. The Department can and does act in this way, but so far only in selected areas. In the *Science and Innovation Strategy* the Department refers to its role in the development of vaccines:

> *2.16 One area in which the Department of Health plays a very particular role in technology development and transfer is in vaccines development. … To support longer term research on vaccines the Department, together with Biotechnology and Biological Sciences Research Council, Medical Research Council and Glaxo Smith Kline, provides support for the Edward Jenner Institute for Vaccine Research.*

Department of Health, 2001m

But this is not its general stance. In the area of vaccines, the Department has had a clear view of its customer role. In other areas, however, such a clear view has not emerged. The Foresight report argues that if the NHS is to be more widely involved in health care development it must reorient itself:

> *from its current reactive stance to be proactive towards the takeup and purchasing of key innovations in order to avoid R&D and other capacity being lost to other countries.*

DTI/OST, 2001, para.14.6

But the issue is not just one of 'lost capacity': the needs of the NHS may also not be served as well as they might be if the Department of Health is not proactive in determining what those needs are and fostering developments to meet them.

This is not to suggest that *all* the impetus for innovation should flow from the public to the private sector – only that there may well be a role in other areas akin to that adopted in vaccine development. But the *Science and Innovation Strategy* paper lacks any intellectual framework within which to set its proposals and to identify what else needs to be done. In particular, it lacks a proper analysis of what the public role should be and how the two main elements of that, support for wealth and support for health, inter-relate. The partnership agreement between the Department of Health and the pharmaceutical industry appears set to fill part of this gap, provided that the Department is active in defining those areas where it believes research is needed. But such gaps are not confined to those where the drug companies have expertise and are willing to engage in joint ventures.

Overview

The health research economy is so complex that it is impossible in a brief review of this kind to determine whether its elements work better as a whole than they did in 1988. On the face of it, substantial progress has been made through the various interlocking procedures described above.

But we have also been able to show that the role of the public sector has not yet been effectively determined. In none of the documents appearing over the past ten or more years has an attempt been made to define it, in the context of the health research economy as a whole. Accordingly, there has been no statement since the Government's response to the 1988 report as to what its view of an effective health research economy would look like. Nor has the Government set out what broad criteria might be used to determine whether or not the changes made within the public domain have improved the working of the whole.

In particular, there has been no attempt to assess whether the public elements of the research economy are contributing to it in those ways which the analysis of Chapter 2 suggested were specific to the role of the State: responding to 'failures' on the part of others. These 'failures' reflect the rules that the other players, commercial and not-for-profit, work under. Our argument suggests that the public role should be either to fill the gaps left by these failures or to devise incentive structures which lead others to do so.

A second concern arises from the threat to diversity stemming from some of the developments referred to here. As noted in Chapter 2, there is a risk that both Government and the scientific community can operate as monopolists in the finance and the production of knowledge. In the long run, science can be seen as a self-correcting process, as can the democratic process. But in the short run, 'market failures' in both finance and production can damage the way the health research economy works. The risk is all the greater if the health research economy becomes less rather than more diverse.

The diversity of the health research economy can be seen as a source of strength – as the Government response to the 1988 report emphasised. No one body can or should attempt to control the entirety of it. But the Government is the only player that can consciously adopt the role of 'system orchestrator'. It has adopted this role in certain areas, particularly in relation to the various public sector players. It has been slower to do so in respect of the private sector's role in the health, rather than the wealth economy.

Chapter 7
Case studies

This chapter takes two subject areas which have a long tradition of science-based research: cancer and Parkinson's disease. It examines how the biases and market failures discussed in earlier chapters affect these two fields. As in the health research field as a whole, there appears to be no clearly defined role for the Department of Health or any overall strategy.

Case studies

In this chapter we take two subject areas and chart how research in these areas has been managed. The first, cancer, is a major cause of mortality, and has attracted significant research funding for 100 years. Parkinson's disease, by contrast, is a degenerative disease affecting a much small number of people. Both, however, appear on the list of conditions mentioned in the 1988 House of Lords report as being under-researched (see p.84). Both attract support from the private not-for-profit sector, as well as public funds, and in both there has been a long tradition of science-based research.

Cancer

Cancer research absorbs a larger share of the health research economy than any other disease. In the framework of this paper we cannot hope to do full justice to the whole of cancer research nor are we qualified to consider its clinical content. Instead we focus on a small number of areas, most of them illuminated by a recent report *Cancer Research: A fresh approach*, from the House of Commons Science and Technology Committee (House of Commons, 2000) and documents published since by the Department of Health.

As the Committee's report revealed, cancer research, like R&D in general, is funded by a pluralist system, the origins of which go back to the beginning of the 20th century with the foundation of the Institute of Cancer Research. Furthermore, from the foundation of the NHS onwards, there have been a series of official reports on how cancer care should be organised. This has meant that, in the field of cancer services, unlike most other parts of the NHS, ideas have been current for decades as to what the role of hospitals and primary care should be. Although the prime focus of these reports has been service delivery, they have also recognised the close links between delivery on the one hand and research and teaching on the other: see the extracts from a report by the Central Health Services Council in the box below.

CANCER CARE AND RESEARCH: EARLY PROPOSALS

The history of attempts to define a strategy towards cancer care and its links with research goes back a long way. In 1949, the Minister of Health issued a paper (Ministry of Health, 1949) stating that a 'cancer service should provide a single organisation to serve a large population of the order of two million to four million'. This service should be structured according to the type of hierarchy which much later documents were to adopt. The cover letter emphasised the need for 'central collection and analysis of records'.

In 1971 a report from the Central Health Services Council, itself building on earlier work, proposed that:

> (iii) *A few comprehensive central cancer organisations should be established which, acting together, would also meet some national needs. These organisations are referred to as 'oncological centres' meaning the hubs from which a cancer service radiate, and places where special facilities and experience would be concentrated (p.24).*
>
> *A framework should be developed to provide research scientists with access to these patients and the clinical specialists in oncology with access to expert research methodology. There would be great advantages to be gained for basic cancer research workers by putting them in touch with a wide range of appropriately trained clinicians with an adequate number of patients suffering from similar tumours under their care who, from a background of experience over the whole tumour range, could concentrate their efforts for reasonable periods of time on one particular problem (p.27).*

> 27. *The close association between fundamental cancer research and the clinical care of patients with cancer is an essential feature of the proposed oncological centres. A research laboratory must therefore*

continued opposite

CANCER CARE AND RESEARCH: EARLY PROPOSALS *continued*

be a key part of each centre. Two factors are considered to be of special importance in this respect:

(i) *the research laboratory must be of sufficient size to provide the 'critical mass' of workers for a reasonably broad multidisciplinary approach in fundamental cancer research, and*

(ii) *the direction of the laboratories must provide facilities for patient-orientated projects irrespective of whether such projects originate from basic research or from clinical practice.*

It is expected that the financing of the cancer research laboratories would be provided largely through the appropriate granting agencies such as the Medical Research Council and the Cancer Research Campaign. The co-ordination of their efforts should be facilitated by the newly formed Cancer Co-ordinating Committee (p.29).

41. *An oncological organisation such as that proposed would need to be based on whatever new regional structure is created for the National Health Service. Its aim would be to:*

(i) *concentrate investigations and treatment into clinical units attracting sufficient patients to improve patient care by allowing experience to be gained of all types of neoplastic disorder*

(ii) *establish focal centres (few in number) to form a framework for a cancer service*

(iii) *encourage internal referral of patients within a group of co-operating hospitals so that each person concerned may have at his disposal the best service available for his need through adequate experience built up within diagnostic, therapeutic, and research units in whatever part of the oncological organisation they may be located*

(iv) *provide a regional co-ordinating information and advice service to cover all general practice and hospital units within the organisation, particularly in relation to those common tumours where there is less need for concentration of patient care*

continued overleaf

CANCER CARE AND RESEARCH: EARLY PROPOSALS *continued*

(v) *break down traditional boundaries both in research departments and in clinical therapeutic disciplines so as to encourage inter-actions at all levels in research, teaching, and clinical practice*

(vi) *concentrate research in groups large enough to allow a flexible multidisciplinary approach*

(vii) *include within such an organisation the provisions at present being made nationally for acute leukaemia, paediatric oncology, and some other rare malignancies* (p.31).

The report also noted the central role of general practitioners in the management of cancer. However, in its 1977 report the Council noted, with regret, that the Department of Health did not have sufficient research funds to allow an external evaluation of the four pilot regional cancer organisations that had been established in the early 1970s.

The Council was disbanded soon afterwards. It was not until the early 1990s that serious efforts to introduce a proper system for the delivery of cancer care and its accompanying research infrastructure began with the London Implementation Group (1993) report on cancer services in London. The Calman Hine committee report followed a few years later (Calman and Hine, 1995). These provided much of the underpinning of the subsequent Cancer Plan (Department of Health, 2000i).

Cancer was one of the areas reviewed following the publication of *Research for Health* (Department of Health, 19991a) and then again in the further tranche of reviews carried out in the second half of the 1990s. It might be expected therefore that research in this area would be well organised and structured against a backcloth of a clear set of views about priorities.

However, the Science and Technology Committee of the House of Commons found a large number of weaknesses (House of Commons, 2000). The most critical were chronic under-funding, totally inadequate infrastructure and a general abdication of responsibility on the part of Government to the not-for-profit sector which, it found, provided the bulk of research funding.

It also found that research was being held back by poor organisation of the delivery of care:

> There is widespread agreement that the poor state of the infrastructure for cancer treatment and research in the NHS is a serious barrier to clinical research. The government must act quickly to address this through investment in the necessary staff, training, equipment and buildings.

House of Commons, 2000, para.91

As the box on pp.172–74 indicates, cancer has been the focus of official reports since the beginning of the NHS and those reports have identified the links between the organisation of the delivery of care and that of research, particularly the proper organisation of records and other infrastructure.

During the 1990s, the first steps were taken at national level to improve the organisation of both care and research. As noted above, cancer was the subject of one of the disease area topic groups set up to advise on research needs by the CRDC. The subsequent report identified 25 priority areas and several other areas which the group thought important, specifically:

- the maintenance of a structure for clinical trials
- the importance of cancer registries
- work on the economics of cancer.

(Department of Health, 1994b, p.9)

While this report was being written, proposals were being prepared for the reorganisation of cancer services in London as part of the work of the London Implementation Group, established after publication of the report of the Tomlinson Inquiry (Tomlinson, 1992). The report from the London Implementation Group (1993) proposed a system of cancer care embodying the notions of specialist centres and a hierarchy of care which had in outline been proposed in earlier reports. Following this report, an expert committee was established to review the national pattern of cancer care and make recommendations for the future pattern of services (Calman and Hine, 1995). The recommendations of the expert group were subsequently adopted as official policy and the process of implementation began.

In 1999 *Strategic Priorities in Cancer Research and Development* was published as one of five topic reports commissioned in 1997. It concluded (Department of Health, 1999d, p.13) that the commissioned programmes which resulted from the 1994 report (Department of Health, 1994b) had produced research which had not been previously funded by other bodies – a clear success for the new arrangements, albeit a limited one. Like the 1994 report, the 1999 report noted improvements in cancer survival rates, but it was also unable to pin down the factors explaining them.[62] It could therefore give no guidance as where it was most important to devote investment in either research or services. However, by the time the Select Committee began its work, there had been no time for the 1999 report to have an impact, whatever its conclusions had been.

The 1999 report did however set out the nature of the cancer research economy. Table 7, opposite, sets out its estimates of spending by some of the main contributors.

These figures do not include spending by the Department of Health/NHS. The Science and Technology Committee obtained the data shown in Table 8, opposite, for these contributions.

As the figures in Table 8 confirm, despite the importance attached to cancer in the national R&D programme, the publicly financed contribution to cancer care was less than that of other main funders – even if the figures presented were correct – and the programme begun as a result of the 1994 review were tiny in relation to the whole.[63] But the Committee did not in fact believe the Government's own figures on cancer research funding:

> *The conviction of many witnesses and of those we met on visits is that most of the NHS R&D funding was disappearing into general support*

---

62. The review drew the following (preliminary) conclusions: '1.11 The Topic Group has concluded that cancer is a massive burden but that some improvements in outcomes for cancer patients have resulted from a wide range of different strategies, probably all of which are likely to continue to contribute to improved outcomes in the foreseeable future. These can be enhanced by effective R&D in the NHS. Basic biomedical research which may lead to novel medical and biological insights and interventions in the medium and long term remains an important area of research carried out by many agencies in this country and abroad, and should be facilitated by the NHS through Partnership arrangements.'

63. See McGeary and Burstein (1999) for a review of US funding of cancer research. In 1997 they estimate that the USA spent some $5 billion on cancer research, of which three-fifths came from the federal budget and a tenth from the non-profit sector.

TABLE 7: ESTIMATED RESEARCH EXPENDITURE 1997/98 (UK CO-ORDINATING COMMITTEE FOR CANCER RESEARCH FUNDING BODIES > £1M/YEAR)

FUNDING BODY	EXPENDITURE (£M)
Imperial Cancer Research Fund	54
Cancer Research Campaign	48.5
Medical Research Council	27*
Leukaemia Research Fund	14.5
Ludwig Institute for Cancer Research	5.6
Institute for Cancer Research	
donations and legacies	5.3
research and academic	61.3
Yorkshire Cancer Research	3.5
Association for International Cancer Research	2.8
Marie Curie	1.5
Tenovus Foundation	1.4

* This figure includes research directly relevant to cancer. It is likely to be an underestimate of the full MRC commitment as it does not include fellowships and studentships and does not take into account the wide range of basic cell biology and genetic research funded by the MRC that may also be relevant to cancer.

Source: Department of Health, 1999d, p.11

TABLE 8: DEPARTMENT OF HEALTH R&D EXPENDITURE ON CANCER, 1998/99

PROGRAMME	EXPENDITURE (£M)
Support for NHS Providers	62.9
Central and Regional Programmes	4.2
Sub-total, NHS Cancer R&D	67.1
Policy Research Programme	2.1
Other[1]	6.3
Total	75.5

1. Department of Health *ad hoc* R&D budgets on radiation, £2.3 million; National Radiological Protection Board, £4.1 million

Source: House of Commons, 2000, p.11

for NHS hospitals and that little of it was actually made available for research purposes. This situation is deeply unsatisfactory.

House of Commons, 2000, para.140

Despite this confusion, it was clear to the Committee that the balance of funding was wrong:

Most UK cancer researchers receive far more support from the research charities and the pharmaceutical industry than they do from the Government. We believe that this imbalance is unhealthy. Notwithstanding the Government's wish to partner and co-operate with cancer research charities, if it does not fund research then the research which it wishes to see will not be done. Cancer research charities cannot and should not be expected to fund research as part of a national strategy. The Government has abdicated its responsibility for cancer research and has by default placed the research agenda in the hands of charities and industry.

House of Commons, 2000, para.145

The Committee recommended an immediate increase in funding of £100 million. That figure was not based on any detailed reasoning: rather it represented an almost visceral response to the situation it found.

The Government responded by promising to match the contribution of the other players. In a subsequent report (House of Commons, 2002), the Committee tried to look further into Government funding. New figures were presented which suggested that total public spending amounted to some £190 million, but the Committee was unimpressed:

In the course of this inquiry we have found the attitude of the Department of Health to the provision on financial facts and figures highly frustrating. We have been forced to ask several times for breakdowns and clarification of spending. We remain to be convinced by some of the figures given. The Department of Health has given no information as to how the totals for those other than for the Department itself were calculated.

House of Commons, 2002, para.11

It therefore concluded that 'there remains at least a suspicion that at least some of the increase in spending is the result of rebadging' (para.12).

More significantly, however, it also concluded that the existing division of roles could not be justified against any set of principles as to what the different contributions should be from the different players in the cancer research economy. Furthermore, it found that the Department of Health was not an 'informed purchaser' despite the wide-ranging conclusions of the 1994 review. As a result, the cancer research economy was biased against those issues which neither part of the private sector was interested in. One such area is the organisation and delivery of services.

The organisation and delivery of care

By the time the Calman Hine committee was at work, it was becoming accepted that proposals for service delivery ought to be based on evidence rather than opinion, even if that opinion was 'well informed'. The official reports prior to the one from the London Implementation Group (1993) had relied entirely on such well-informed professional opinion. The Calman Hine committee tried, but was unable, to find a great deal of evidence bearing on its proposals, particularly around the key question of the benefits of specialisation by individual clinicians and by hospitals.[64] The NHS Cancer Plan (Department of Health, 2000i) largely followed the proposals of the expert committee (Calman Hine) without any further substantive discussion of the underlying knowledge base.

However, the 1999 cancer review had pointed out that the links between the organisation and delivery of care and better outcomes is not clear. In its conclusions it states that:

> *gaps in evidence which are critical to the planning of service developments are prominent. … They relate to many aspects of diagnosis and treatment.*

Department of Health, 1999d, p.25

The NHS Cancer Plan was therefore an 'act of faith', albeit one which had widespread professional support. But such support is not necessarily enough. During 2000 and 2001 a series of papers were published in the

---

64. In general the evidence supports a higher degree specialisation by clinicians (and teams) in individual cancer sites. However, good results have also been obtained by medium-sized hospitals in which the clinicians work within agreed protocols.

Lancet and elsewhere on the benefits of breast cancer screening. At the very least, these papers showed that the issue is not clear-cut. Nevertheless, official statements about the UK screening programme continue to assert its value in saving lives.

Proposals for a National Cancer Research Institute

The House of Commons Science and Technology Committee concluded that there was no co-ordination in the cancer research economy. To fill this gap the Committee proposed that a National Cancer Research Institute should be established, with a wide range of functions (see box opposite).

It went on to argue that:

> *The National Cancer Research Institute should operate at arm's length from Government under the authority of its own Royal Charter, accountable to Parliament through the Minister for Science. We do not envisage it as a large organisation but as a small authority with a physical existence. It should not have its own intramural research programme, other than through the cancer registries, nor should it be based in an existing research facility.*
>
> House of Commons, 2000, para.56

While the Institute was to provide the organisational framework for developing cancer research, the Committee proposed that: 'a cancer research strategy should become an integral part of the National Cancer Plan' (House of Commons, 2000).

The Government accepted the main thrust of the Committee's analysis. Its response acknowledged that:

> *there are weaknesses in the overall pattern of cancer research. High level strategic planning and coordination has been insufficient.*
>
> Department of Health, 2000c, para.6

The Cancer Plan confirms that the National Cancer Research Institute is to be established, adding that:

> *One of the key tasks of [the Institute] will be to co-ordinate research into cancer genetics funded by government, charities and*

PROPOSED ROLES FOR A NATIONAL CANCER RESEARCH INSTITUTE

*We recommend the creation of a new National Cancer Research
Institute to set national research priorities and to co-ordinate and fund
cancer research in the UK. It should:*

*Co-ordinate cancer research in the UK by developing a cancer research
strategy and identifying gaps in research funding; Ensuring
integration and complementarity between the Calman Hine cancer
care networks and research networks ...*

Set priorities for clinical research;

*Set and implement priorities for cancer registration strategy
by managing and funding the National Cancer Registry, and
co-ordinating and funding regional cancer registries;*

*Determine and set out the case for appropriate levels of Government
funding for cancer research;*

*Receive all Government funds for cancer research and allocate them
to extra-mural research programmes and projects, on the basis of
appropriate mechanisms of peer review;*

*Make available assistance in peer review to charities funding cancer
research;*

*Produce and maintain Good Clinical Practice guidelines and oversee
adherence to them;*

Provide guidance and co-ordinate training for oncologists;

*Issue and maintain guidance, subject to regular review, on the
diagnosis of malignancy in general practice;*

*Co-ordinate the provision of appropriate tumour, tissue and serum
depositories for cancer research; and*

Communicate with the public on issues related to cancer.

(House of Commons, 2000, pp.19–20)

*industry. This country should be at the forefront of this rapidly
developing area.*

Department of Health, 2000i, para.10.9

The NHS Cancer Plan also confirms some of the criticisms made by the
Committee about the organisation of cancer research:

> *there are weaknesses in the cancer research endeavours in this
> country. There has been insufficient high-level strategic planning
> and co-ordination between the different funding partners. The
> infrastructure for clinical research has been inadequate and there
> has been insufficient support for specific areas of research which
> could lead to important improvements in service delivery.*

Department of Health, 2000i, para.10.4

Against this background it is not surprising that the Government accepted
the Committee's main recommendations.

> *10.7 ... the Director of NHS Research and Development and the
> National Cancer Director have been asked to work with all those
> involved in the funding and delivery of cancer research to come
> forward with definitive proposals for a National Cancer Research
> Institute (NCRI). The NCRI will be a partnership between government,
> the voluntary sector and the private sector. The Institute will have
> strategic oversight of the cancer research conducted in this country. It
> will take the lead in identifying areas where further research initiatives
> are needed and most likely to lead to progress.*

Department of Health, 2000i

Thus by the middle of 2002, the process of building up machinery
designed to develop an effective cancer research economy had begun.
But the situation as the Science and Technology Committee found it was
far from satisfactory. In particular:

- Despite nearly ten years of effort and, despite the excellence of
  individual parts of it, cancer research appears disorganised.
- Some of the essential underpinnings, identified years previously, are
  not in place.
- As the recent *ad hoc* injection of funds into prostate cancer research
  indicates, the existing allocation within cancer research has not
  been effective.

- The underlying features of the new way of delivering care remain largely unsupported by research evidence.
- The roles of the various players and the interfaces between them remain to be determined.
- A strategic view of research needs is still awaited.

The Government's response to the Committee and the limited statements in the Cancer Plan reflect an acceptance that, despite all the efforts of the

---

RESEARCH INTO PROSTATE CANCER

The Cancer Plan accepted the need for more research, but was very unspecific as to what that research should consist of, with the exception of research into prostate cancer. As it happens, as the Plan was being developed, a campaign developed, led (if that is the word) by the *Daily Mail*, for more research into prostate cancer. In due course, the Government announced a prostate cancer programme. In March 2000, the Public Health Minister announced £1 million funding 'for urgent research studies into prostate cancer' (Department of Health, 2000h).

At around the same time the *Daily Mail* put up a similar figure.[65] Further increases were subsequently announced for 2003/04. When announcing these increases, the Minister accepted that:

> Over 10,000 men die from prostate cancer every year yet little research has been carried out around the world into early detection of the disease as well as the best treatment and prevention methods.

Department of Health 2000h

This suggests that even within the clinical field worldwide there was a serious imbalance in current efforts as between different types of cancer. This is a particularly striking case, given the high level of incidence of prostate cancer: almost any criterion for allocating research resources should have resulted in this cancer receiving substantial support.[66]

---

65. At about the same time the author received a 'begging letter' from a hospital-based research group seeking funds for prostate cancer research.

66. Some of the evidence to the House of Commons Science and Technology Committee comes from individuals or groups who argue that their particular cancer has had low priority in both research and clinical developments.

previous decades, the balance of research was not right. It also implies that the fundamentals – research infrastructure, clinical trial organisation and cancer registries – were not in place.

Given that cancer has been a national priority for a decade, the obvious question to raise is: Why had these weaknesses not been addressed before?

Reasons behind the failure to create a framework for research

As the box on pp.172–4 records, some of these weaknesses had been identified years before. A number of expert committees had attempted to take a strategic view of cancer research, while others had addressed the delivery of cancer care, and models of cancer care had been published. But until the implementation of Calman-Hine began, there had been no effective central initiative. It is tempting therefore to ascribe the failure to procure high level co-ordination to a failure of machinery, which the measures proposed by the Government in its response to the Science and Technology Committee will begin to address.

That explanation has some surface validity: the 'cancer research economy' is enormously complex, as it embodies all the characteristics set out above of the wider health research economy, and there has never been any agency spanning all the relevant actors even within the public sector. While the NHS presents a monolithic face to outsiders, inside it appears fragmented. And while the central role has appeared too powerful in recent years, as seen from the perspective of the NHS as a whole, it has, in critical areas such as service design, been weak (see, for example, Harrison, 2001).

But that failure is in turn explicable in terms of other, underlying, factors. Many of the weaknesses identified stem, on the one hand, from a failure at the centre to appreciate the requirements for effective research and, on the other, from the essentially individualistic culture of medicine and of clinical research. Both have militated against taking an effective overview of the whole. Thus even where, as with the 1994 and the 1999 reviews, an attempt was made to take an overview, the result was fragmentary and partial.

Such fragmentation persists in the NHS Cancer Plan which, though more or less comprehensive, does not provide a framework which demonstrates the linkages between its various elements. Nor has it managed to provide what the Select Committee suggested: a systematic research plan.

The failure here seems as much an intellectual as an administrative one. What the Plan and all the other documents we have drawn on in this section lack is a coherent intellectual framework for considering 'the whole'. As we noted above, by far the greater proportion of publicly funded R&D follows in the clinical research tradition of focusing on narrowly defined issues – the HTA makes a virtue of this. But while this focus is the *sine qua non* of progress, at the same time it is insufficient. In cancer, as for other diseases, there is a need to consider how various interventions relate to each other. To some degree, this point is acknowledged in the way that clinical research is designed. For example, in the case of breast cancer, a great deal of work has been aimed at determining the right sequence and combination of different treatments.

But taking the field as a whole, there has been no attempt to consider how the various main interventions relate to each other. As the 1994 report noted and the 1999 report reaffirmed, survival rates have improved, but it is not clear what the relative contributions to that result has been. The same is true of the changes resulting from the Calman Hine proposals. As Kerr and Edwards point out:

> *implementation of the regional cancer plan can be seen as a large-scale public health experiment in which we are testing the hypothesis that a linked, multi-discplinary cancer service that depends on inter-trust cooperation will improve our cancer survival figures.*

> Kerr and Edwards, 2000, p.42

As this indicates, the reorganisation of cancer care represents an enormous gamble. But, even if survival rates improve, it will not be clear which of the many changes involved have been significant.

We conclude therefore that although the case for a National Cancer Research Institute is *prima facie* strong, given the evident weaknesses in existing arrangements, institutional change must be accompanied by intellectual development as well. Otherwise the risk is that results will continue to be fragmentary and disjointed. This is the central weakness identified by the topic review of ageing (Department of Health, 1999c) which considered that a new way of conceptualising research requirements was needed – what it termed the 'laboratory approach'.

But what that means in practice remains to be worked out. A regional cancer system or a local system of care for elderly people can be a 'laboratory' in name only: none of the control requirements applies. Quite rightly the NHS Cancer Plan is focusing on those areas such as speed of access and the condition of the capital assets required to deliver care where current shortfalls are obvious.

But if, as the Science and Technology Committee urged, a research plan should be at the centre of the Cancer Plan, much more than a wish list of projects is required.[67] Rather, some integrating framework is required within which the potential value of improvements in particular parts of the cancer care system can be assessed (including patients and carers as part of that system). The framework should also enable the assessment of the interaction of parts of the system and should define what monitoring and tracking arrangements are needed to provide the basis for such assessments (see Mulligan, 2000, for a further discussion).

Parkinson's disease

Parkinson's disease is often cited as a seminal case of the application of science to treat a medical condition (West, 1991). Initially, the symptoms of Parkinson's disease – tremor, muscular rigidity and slowness of movement – were shown in 1915 to reflect a dysfunction in the *substantia nigra* region of the brain. In the 1950s, it was discovered that this collection of nerve cells produced and stored the chemical dopamine. Damage to the *substantia nigra* caused deficiency of dopamine, which led to the symptoms of Parkinsonism. In 1957 it was suggested that the metabolic precursor of dopamine – levodopa – might be used in the treatment of the disease.

---

67. The need for new thinking has also been put by Michael Baum, himself a distinguished clinician: 'It is time for a new start in the "war" against cancer. The contemporary paradigm served its purpose and we require more innovative approaches to the understanding and treatment of the disease.' (Baum, 2000, p.47).

Parkinson's disease was the first example of a neurological disease consistently correlated with a deficiency in a specific neurotransmitter (dopamine). ... [The treatment with levodopa] marked the first attempt to cure a brain disease by exogenously administering a neurotransmitter precursor.

West, 1991, pp.17–18

Treatment with levodopa remains the principal and most effective treatment for Parkinson's disease, and many of the treatment advances have come from additional drugs working either in parallel with levodopa, or to delay the need for the use of levodopa (which has its own damaging side-effects). However, a number of new forms of treatment have also developed over the last two decades (Larkin, 1999).

'Glutamate inhibitors' and 'neuroprotective therapy' are examples of treatments which aim to slow or even halt the progression of the disease itself. Deep brain stimulation for patients with advanced Parkinson's disease seeks to work by a 'jamming' process or by activating inhibitory systems. Continuous dopaminergic stimulation is an alternative for advanced-state Parkinson's disease for those with severe levodopa side-effects. Most recently there have been the now widely publicised implants from aborted foetuses, or in the future from embryo-derived stem cell lines that can be multiplied indefinitely and used to produce standardised 'pure' dopaminergic neurons.

The National Research Register contains information on research which is being funded by, or of interest to, the NHS at any given point in time. It is not necessarily comprehensive, relying on the people doing research to submit their activities. It includes projects funded via the HTA programme and other national programmes.

Table 9, overleaf, shows that Government funding is clearly dominated by the HTA grant for the multi-centre trial of various Parkinson's drugs. Other projects are financed by a variety of institutions, as well as benefiting from the R&D Support for Science funding streams. The other main arm of State funding is the MRC which spent £1.4 million in 1998/99 (personal communication, Ruth Carleton, MRC). This expenditure is often in collaboration with charities or other streams of funding from Government.

TABLE 9: CURRENT, ONGOING PROJECTS ON PARKINSON'S DISEASE ON THE NATIONAL RESEARCH REGISTER

INTERVENTION	METHODOLOGY	FUNDING	SETTING	COMPLETION DATE
Ropinirole, for patients with early PD	Double blind, multi-centre, l-dopa controlled	SmithKline Beecham	Southend Hospital NHS Trust	2002
Aetiology of UCH-LI	Laboratory study	PD Society, £60,000	Institute of Child Health	2003
Accuracy of computer-based diagnostic techniques	Cross-sectional study; 50 people with PD, 50 age-matched control	Movement Disorders Trust, £500 (*sic*)	Broadgreen Hospital NHS Trust	2002
Multi-centre comparison of efficacy and cost-effectiveness of various PD drugs	Randomised trial using patient questionnaires and hospital data	HTA programme, £1,000,000	University of Birmingham/Queen Elizabeth Hospital Clinical Trials Unit	2010
			Powys Health Care NHS Trust	2002
			Walsgrave Hospitals NHS Trust	2009
			Royal Wolverhampton Hospitals NHS Trust	2006
Assessment of the risk of falling, and prediction of future trends	Descriptive, prospective study	British Geriatrics Society, £1,944	North Tyneside General Hospital	2001
Development of improved electrical stimulation system for advanced PD	n/a	PD Society, amount n/a	Oxford Radcliffe Hospital NHS Trust	2003
Investigation of the effect of lesioning and deep brain surgery	n/a	Medtronic Ltd, amount n/a	Royal Hallamshire Hospital University of Sheffield	2001
Diagnostic value of iron deposition	n/a, but using MRI scans	PD Society, £73,371	Royal Hallamshire Hospital	2002
To aid clinical management of visual hallucinations in patients with PD	n/a	PD Society, £10,000	Royal Hallamshire Hospital	2002
Trial of anti-depressants in PD	RCT	PD Society and SmithKline Beecham, £60,000	South Birmingham Mental Health NHS Trust	2003

PD = Parkinson's disease

There are no figures available for the contribution of the for-profit private sector as a whole. The principal voluntary sector contributor is the Parkinson's Disease Society of the UK, which spent approximately £1.0 million in 1999 on medical or welfare research (Parkinson's Disease Society of the UK, 1999). The table below shows expenditure on various categories of project (all current projects expected to end in 2002 or later).

TABLE 10: EXPENDITURE ON PARKINSON'S DISEASE RESEARCH PROJECTS

GENERAL CATEGORY OF RESEARCH	RESEARCH CENTRE	TYPE OF RESEARCH METHODOLOGY	GRANT	TIME SCALE	END DATE
MR: Alpha-Synuclein in Lewy bodies and Lewy Neurites	Brain Repair Centre, Cambridge	Lab research	£124,485	3 years	2002
	UCL	Lab research	£98,875	2 years	2002
	Royal Free and UCL	Lab research	£115,625	3 years	2002
	Lancaster University	Lab research	£176,489	3 years	2004
MR: Symptoms, physical and cognitive	Brain Repair Centre, Cambridge	Observational study to determine sub-types of PD	£162,258	3 years	2003
	King's College London	Observational study of time-use	£107,490	3 years	2004
MR: Dopamine	King's College London	Lab study	£74,412	18 months	2002
	Imperial College and Charing Cross Hospital	Lab study	£106,473	2 years	2002
	University of Edinburgh	Lab study	£58,916	2 years	2002
	King's College London	Lab study	£97,847	3 years	2002
MR: Drug treatment and processing	University of Sheffield	Lab study	£44,887	18 months	2002
MR: Genes	Imperial College School of Medicine	Lab study	£133,199	2 years	2002

continued overleaf

TABLE 10: EXPENDITURE ON PARKINSON'S DISEASE RESEARCH PROJECTS *continued*

GENERAL CATEGORY OF RESEARCH	RESEARCH CENTRE	TYPE OF RESEARCH METHODOLOGY	GRANT	TIME SCALE	END DATE
MR: Surgical treatments	Imperial College	Lab study	£133,952	3 years	2003
	Brain Repair Centre, Cambridge	Lab study	£117,102	3 years	2002
	Brain Repair Centre, Cambridge	Lab study	£88,401	3 years	2003
Joint MR and WR: fatigue	King's College London, Dept Psychology and Inst. of Psychiatry	Lab study	n/a	n/a	2003
WR: Care and the multidisciplinary team	University of Birmingham	Delphi study and protocol design for RCT of occupational therapy	£49,765	1 year	2003
WR: Complementary therapies	De Montfort University, Leicester	Qualitative assessments of complementary therapies	£4,950	2 years	2002
	University of Exeter	Test practicality of full RCT	£10,000	1 year	n/a
WR: Miscellaneous	King's and St Thomas' Dental Institute	non-randomised controlled trial (n=20) of dental implants	£24,975	3 years	2004

Notes: MR = Medical Research; WR = Welfare Research; PD = Parkinson's disease

'Welfare research' is defined by the Society as 'all research relating to Parkinson's disease which does not aim to find a cause or cure for the disease or test the efficacy of drugs or surgery in the control of symptoms'.

It is difficult to draw any firm conclusions from these data alone. Parkinson's clearly receives far less funding than cancer, but given the numbers affected by each condition, that may seem reasonable enough. But it remains the case that there can still be a mismatch on a like-for-like basis, taking the average expenditure per person with the disease. For example, in a recent debate in the USA about its National Institutes of Health, one commentator listed the Institutes' expenditure per head for a number of diseases: $2143 per head for AIDS, $200 for breast cancer, $81 for Alzheimer's and $20 for diabetes (Greenberg, 1997). Unfortunately, equivalent figures are not readily available in the UK, but it is likely that similar disparities will prevail.

The response from the National Institutes of Health was that deciding on research priorities was far more complex than this. Diabetes, for example, though incurable, can be managed very successfully, allowing people to lead normal lives. One might argue, therefore, that it has a lower priority. They also argued that they have learned that the most significant and rapid advances are likely to occur when new findings expand experimental possibilities.

In other words, some diseases may be more likely provide a 'return' on research than others, because of the general state of knowledge about those diseases. Furthermore, and citing Parkinson's disease as an example, it argued that specific research projects are often complemented by the much larger number of projects devoted to basic science, such as nerve-cell biology, dopamine metabolism and neurodegeneration, that have obvious implications for the future treatment of the disease, albeit with potentially difficult ethical consequences.

In the case of Parkinson's disease, the weaknesses seem much less salient than those identified in the cancer field. The main issue has been to find viable research approaches. Fundamental work at the 'pure' end of the spectrum may provide what is needed to open these up – as indeed the recent development with stem cells suggests. In other words lack of resources and poor organisation have not been the main obstacle to progress, but rather, as with cancer three to four decades ago, a lack of clear avenues for research and slow progress along those which have been identified.

Nevertheless it is striking that there is no Government strategy for research directed at this disease. One is awaited, however: the proposed national service framework for neurological conditions is due to be published in 2004 and that is expected to contain research proposals which may fill the gap.

Overview

The examples considered here reflect very different circumstances. Nevertheless, both the areas considered lack a strategy and in neither is the role of the Department of Health/NHS clear. In neither case is it possible to see beyond a national collection of projects to a view or set of views as to who should be doing what.

In the case of Parkinson's disease it will be some time before such a view emerges. In the case of cancer, the Government's response to the House of Commons Science and Technology Committee report and the formation of the National Cancer Research Institute may well provide the strategic view missing so far, although, if our analysis above is correct, more is required than mere machinery. The very concept of a research strategy has yet to be given substantive meaning in the fields considered here or indeed any other.

Chapter 8

The health research economy in context

This chapter takes a broader view of the changing context of the health research economy. The public is increasingly sceptical of authority, whether professional, scientific or political. This sets a new agenda for policy development: how to involve the public in a dialogue with experts about science policy making.

8 The health research economy in context

The policy developments described in Chapters 3 to 7 can be seen as a sustained attempt to control the provider interest in determining what research should be done and how it should be done. Although these processes have also aimed to involve users in determining priorities, this has been at a very modest level: essentially they remain professionally driven. Many of the assumptions of research providers, research funders and their advisers are held in common. The most fundamental of these is that the knowledge produced by research can be relied on as a basis for action – in the present context, medical and other clinical interventions, including public health policies.

The House of Lords 1988 report, like our own analysis up to this point, assumed that knowledge can be produced and used in an uncontentious way. The health care research economy may be organised better to produce more of it, or more of the right kinds, and biases may be addressed so as to improve its contribution to overall welfare. But our argument has progressed without questioning whether, even under ideal organisational and financial conditions, the knowledge it produces can be considered unequivocally a 'true' reflection of the world, which, once gained, it is the task of professionals to use for the benefit of patients. As we noted in the Introduction, the assumption that it is has been the foundation of medical professional authority for the best part of a century.

This simple schema ignores some fundamental issues. In particular it assumes that we can have complete confidence about the pronouncements of science or any other field of professional enquiry, and hence that once knowledge is produced, the main requirement is to ensure that it is rapidly implemented. But as the first part of this chapter shows, such a high degree of confidence is unattainable. In the second part, therefore, we consider some of the implications of these limitations. Where uncertainty is endemic, it can be difficult for society to manage and use such knowledge as is produced. The question, in short, is: Can we cope with uncertainty? In the final section we consider briefly some of the broader issue of social accountability which this discussion raises.

Limitations

We have implicitly assumed that the health research economy produces knowledge of 'what works' and what does not – knowledge which can then be applied to promoting health and welfare through the delivery of health care and public health measures. The authority of health professionals and of Government when making decisions on the safety of measures outside the health arena or measures within it, such as immunisation programmes, rests on the assumption, largely unquestioned until recently, that both the individual professional and the Government machine possess a reliable knowledge base and one which vastly exceeds what the individual, patient or citizen, can command.

The partial and provisional nature of scientific knowledge

The developments described in this study serve to underline the partial nature of the knowledge which health professionals possess.[68] The biases discussed throughout the earlier chapters reflect the fact that both the producers of knowledge and its professional and official users possess mental blinkers which may serve to increase the acuity with which they perceive what is immediately in front of them, but which prevent them from seeing the larger picture.[69] These mental blinkers may be reinforced by the various sets of incentives discussed in Chapter 2 and Chapter 6, which lead to overemphasis of particular pieces of knowledge and neglect of others.

---

68. For a wider discussion see, for example, Trinder (2000). In particular: 'Research is an inherently political process. The tendency of the evidence-based practice movement has been to respond to this by trying to eliminate bias by technical means and further refinements of this process to produce a somewhat false sense of certainty. Fuller attention to the issues and outcomes of concern to consumers will help. Just as important is a greater degree of reflexivity amongst researchers, reviewers and practitioners to think about what assumptions about the world are taken for granted and what questions and answers are not addressed or precluded by particular pieces of research or particular research designs' (p.237).

69. This point is made in Stowe (1989) and Swales (1997).

The particular pieces of knowledge possessed by health professionals may be valid, i.e. obtained by means which would pass the test of peer review and replicability by others, but unless the total picture into which they fit is as well understood, they may be given greater weight than they deserve.

Although biases of this kind are important, they are not the only reason why the knowledge produced by the health research economy is open to question. However carefully science proceeds, its results are always subject to correction from later findings and hence are always provisional, even if they treated in practice as being 'certain'. The history of medicine displays many examples of the 'certain' proving to be wrong and, while many such changes may be put down to the primitive nature of medical science up to the Second World War, there are many examples since, of which Thalidomide is the classic case.

Ironically, recent attempts to improve the scientific underpinnings of clinical practice have served to reveal the partial and provisional nature of the knowledge on which the health care system rests. The development of evidence-based medicine, supported by processes such as those employed by the HTA programme, has served to underline the fact that much clinical practice has been based on opinion and that in many areas the studies required to determine issues of clinical significance have not been carried out. So while the HTA programme and the similar procedures used by NICE focus on a range of issues of clinical importance and bring to bear on them whatever evidence exists, they cannot produce evidence if it is not there – at least not rapidly.

As things currently stand, NICE does not have access to what would have to be a very substantial research budget to make good the gaps its investigations reveal. The limits of the available evidence are even greater in the broader areas such as hospital configuration and access to elective care, which require analysis drawing on a wide range of evidence from different disciplines.

Nevertheless, the development of evidence-based medicine which uses systematic reviews of the evidence does offer some reassurance to patients that practice is well supported. These procedures typically rely on a hierarchy of research methodologies for understanding whether interventions are the most effective:

- The randomised control trial, preferably 'double blind' stands at the top.
- Next come non-randomised or 'observational' studies such as case control or cohort studies.
- Then there is qualitative research such as interviews or 'participant observation' where quantification is difficult.
- Finally there is research led by an individual practitioner, focusing on the clinician's own experience and practice deriving from the patient–doctor relationship, which is more anecdotal and personal.

But this hierarchy is less powerful than it may seem. It may not always be possible to apply the 'gold-standard' RCT: it may be ethically inappropriate or impossible to arrange, particularly where health care systems are concerned as opposed to specific interventions.[70] But even when more narrowly defined interventions are concerned, the issue of transferability arises. Although reviews of evidence are now conducted in ways which are highly self-conscious about what is good evidence and what is not, no methodology can guarantee reliability when the results are translated into clinical practice (see Swales, 1997).

The methods underpinning evidence-based practice are based on populations not individuals. The very strength of the RCT is, looked at from another angle, that of the individual patient, a critical weakness. This point has been reinforced by the claims arising from the genome project, which suggest that treatments in future will be personalised in the light of the individual's genetic make-up, thereby underlining the limitations of existing approaches.

As Tanenbaum put in nearly a decade ago:

> *Uncertainty is inherent in medical practice because patients present individual and complex medical circumstances. Physicians can never be certain how to transpose a biomedical theory or a clinical research finding to a particular case.*

Tanenbaum, 1993, p.1269

---

70. Furthermore the more rigid the rules of evidence the harder it is to demonstrate certain kinds of causal connections. According to Ewald (2000): 'When standards of evidence are set too high, scientific rigor declines. It is easy to recognize this problem when the standards are set so high they can never be met. If, for example, scientists demanded experimental demonstration of humans evolving from apes, the hypothesis could never be accepted. This too-high standard of evidence would have sapped the rigor of scientific inquiry into human origins.'

The same point is made by many others. Sweeney and colleagues, for example, argue that:

> clinical significance attempts to measure the potential impact of the research [but] it applies only to populations or groups of patients. ... There still remains the difficulty of transporting such population-derived information to the individual person who may not enter the consulting room with a discrete one-dimensional problem.

> Sweeney *et al.*, 1998, p.134

And even when service delivery appears to be solidly founded on reliable research, it may not in fact be so. The recent debates about the value of breast cancer screening illustrate this clearly. Screening programmes have been in place for more than a decade in most developed countries, but recent reviews (Gotzsche and Olsen, 2000) have suggested that they are not beneficial, in part because of methodological weaknesses in what appeared to be 'best practice' studies, leading the *Lancet* to conclude that:

> At present, there is no reliable evidence from large randomised trials to support screening mammography programmes.

> Horton, 2001

Since that article was published, evidence supporting both the sceptics and the proponents of screening has continued to appear.

The difficulties of capturing complexity

More fundamentally, many of the issues research needs to address are too complex for any existing research methodology (Wilson and Holt, 2001). As Plsek and Greenhalgh put it:

> We all know from experience that the management of clinical problems is rarely simple. Yet most of us were taught about and tend to adopt a mental model of the human body as a machine and illness as due to malfunction of its parts. Such linear models drive us to break down clinical care into ever smaller divisions and to express with great accuracy and precision the intervention to be undertaken for each malfunction.

> Complexity science suggests an alternative model – that illness (and health) results from complex, dynamic, and unique interactions

between different components of the overall system. Effective clinical decision making requires a holistic approach that accepts unpredictability and builds up subtle emergent forces within the overall system.

Plsek and Greenhalgh, 2001, p.688

The complexity of systems of health care delivery (see Chapter 4) means that research focusing on any one part runs the risk that its findings will be overturned by changes in the wider setting or, indeed, by other interventions acting on a different part of the system[71] or by changes in personal behaviour.[72]

As noted in Chapter 4, reviews of research requirements have identified approaches which aim to take account of the context in which interventions take place and the interactions between them. But these have not yet been reflected in new forms of research designed to produce useable results, allowing for 'systems' effects. For example, a recent review of the evidence relating to the effects on health of improvements in housing concluded that:

The lack of evidence linking housing to health may be attributable to pragmatic difficulties with housing studies. ... A holistic approach is

---

71. See Hess (1997): 'The first problem is that RCTs tend to focus on single agents or small groups of agents' (p.189) ... 'The magic-bullet strategy is counterproductive to the advancement of cancer therapy. Much of the magic-bullet strategy is driven by the financial necessity of developing a patentable agent that will return a profit on the investments needed to obtain FDA approval for use of a substance as a cancer drug, and of covering the marketing costs of the drug. Furthermore, as Michael Culbert mentioned, a Cartesian research culture values research strategies that break down natural substances into component parts and then test them individually. Once broken down, substances are then combined in very small groups, for example as chemotherapy cocktails. The result is, as John Boik recognized, a painstaking slow pace of research. In contrast, many of the members of the ACCT community emphasize synergy among natural products that are not broken down into constituent compounds and that may act through a variety of biochemical mechanisms' (p.200). Hess makes a number of equally important points.

72. See Trinder (2000), in particular: 'There are major areas where evidence is lacking, questions about the extent to which evidence can be trusted (meta-analysis), questions about the narrowness of evidence and narrowness of outcomes. In some areas certainty is more founded, whilst in other areas, beyond the biological, the search for certainty poses considerable dangers in inherently complex and uncertain worlds. Whilst evidence is potentially helpful it is important not to be seduced into an unwarranted sense of security' (p.237).

needed that recognises the multifactorial and complex nature of poor housing and deprivation. Large scale studies that investigate the wider social context of housing interventions are required.

Thomson *et al.*, 2001, p.187

In the absence of such studies, it is not clear what weight should be attached to results bearing on parts of such systems. Nowhere is this more evident than in those areas where personal behaviour, particularly regarding diet, is deemed important to good health. The public is continually bombarded with research findings about, for example, the links between eating or other behaviour and cancer which often appear contradictory. An *Observer* editorial (17 February 2002) reflected this confusion: 'Every day new tales of unlikely health advice. Fruit and veg cause cancer! Apples rot your teeth! Sun good for you! Sleep kills!'

Most of these findings are based on tightly focused studies of particular relationships between disease and the intake of particular foods or other specific factors. They do not, even to the experts themselves, form part of a coherent picture of 'how things work', taking the interaction of all the relevant factors into account. As McKinlay and Marceau put it:

Risk factor epidemiology generally focuses on the somewhat isolated contribution of one factor while overlooking competing influences from other levels of analysis causality. Although the 'discovery' of new risk factors creates an illusion of progress, we do not know how much any one factor contributes to the total explanation, and whether modification of that risk factor would appreciably alter the prevalence of the condition.

McKinlay and Marceau, 2000, p.757

Public loss of confidence in decision makers

More sceptical views of science as a whole

These methodological issues may not concern the general public directly – although the continuous stream of reports identifying links between diet and cancer or other illnesses most probably does. However, outstanding 'failures' such as Thalidomide and BSE and events outside medicine such as the Government's response to foot and mouth disease have made it clear to all that the confidence which the knowledge base appears to offer to policy making is in fact unjustified.[73] Assurances offered 'with total confidence' turn out to be based on limited evidence and have to be modified or even overturned in the light of subsequent findings. Not surprisingly, there are signs that such events have resulted in a loss of confidence in the overall scientific enterprise from which many such developments stem – but which have also produced unequivocal gains in other areas.

A recent report from the House of Lords Select Committee on Science and Technology put it this way:

> *Society's relationship with science is in a critical phase. Science today is exciting, and full of opportunities. Yet public confidence in scientific advice to Government has been rocked by BSE; and many people are uneasy about the rapid advance of areas such as biotechnology and IT – even though for everyday purposes they take science and technology for granted. This crisis of confidence is of great importance both to British society and to British science.*

House of Lords, 2000b, Introduction

The report is in part based on survey evidence carried out by organisations concerned about the impact of public opinion on the future development of British science. The table opposite presents results from one such survey.

In only one of these subject areas does confidence seem to have improved, with fewer people now agreeing that science makes their lives change too fast. In all the other areas, the trend can be interpreted as one of weakening confidence. Also, it is not reassuring that less than half of those polled believe that science's benefits outweigh its costs.[74]

Why this more explicit emergence of the uncertainties of science and the risks attached to scientific developments seems to be taking place now is a moot point. It may be linked to greater democracy forcing complex

---

73. A *New Scientist* editorial (22/29 December 2001) on the public's attitude to science concluded: 'society at large no longer sees science as the deliverer of simple facts and truths, and no longer unthinkingly accepts scientists' vision of the future. But if blind faith has given way to intelligent scepticism that can only be a good thing.'

74. This phenomenon is not confined to this country, see *Financial Times* (2001).

TABLE 11: PUBLIC ATTITUDES TO SCIENCE

Subject	% Agreeing	
	2000	1996
Science and technology are making our lives healthier, easier and more comfortable.	67	73
In general scientists want to make life better for the average person.	67	–
Because of science, engineering and technology there will be more opportunities for the next generation.	77	–
We depend too much on science and not enough on faith.	38	40
It is important to know about science in my daily life.	59	51
Even if it brings no immediate benefits, scientific research which advances the frontiers of knowledge is necessary and should be supported by the Government.	72	–
Science makes our lives change too fast.	44	53
The benefits of science are greater than the harmful effects.	43	45

Source: DTI/OST/Wellcome Trust (2000)

debates into the open, or to the growth in the use of the Internet and the access it provides to those holding alternative views of scientific progress. Perhaps it is even linked to the scale of certain scientific ambitions – and the misjudgements that accompany them – as we embark on exploring the universe on the one hand and the building blocks of life on the other, both ever more removed from the terms of everyday human experience. Whatever the reasons, the view of science as providing certain and objective knowledge is breaking down and, with it, the original basis of the 'authority' of medicine.

Challenges from a better-informed public

At the same time, the authority of medicine has been attacked from another angle. In recent years the notion of partnership between patients and professionals has come to the fore for a number of reasons. It began with the recognition that choosing the 'best' course of treatment should involve an exchange of information between patient and professional about the implications of different interventions. There has also been a growing realisation that the patient's compliance with whatever course of treatment is chosen is critical. Most recently, the concept of the expert patient has arisen: that the patient may, in some respects, have a greater understanding of his or her own condition and the impact of interventions upon it than the professional. As Muir Gray has put it:

> The parent who has a child with a rare metabolic disease who happens to have had a scientific education will be able to find, read, and understand a paper about the gene definition in Nature, whereas most clinicians would be out of their depth with such a paper. Furthermore, as patients learn that know-how is as important as knowledge and that many clinicians do not have the know-how of managing chronic disease, they will share know-how with one another.

Muir Gray, 1999, p.1552

Patients or carers have been supported by the greater availability of information via the Internet, which has enabled some to be more expert in professional opinion on their illness than their professional advisers.[75] According to Edwards and Elwyn:

> While most professionals do not understand or have access to these modern information technologies, or simply lack sufficient time to familiarize themselves with the Internet, consumers have all the time in the world to search the Internet for relevant information.

Edwards and Elwyn, 2001, p.295

---

75. See, for example, Hess (1999): 'Although empirically grounded to some extent, the transmission model is inadequate because it misses a key component in the public understanding of science: the ability of segments of the public to reconstruct science, that is, to develop their own independent interpretations of official scientific knowledge and their own uses for existing technologies (or, in the medical world, therapies). Consequently, social scientists have develop an alternative "reconstruction" model that replaces the transmission, or diffusion, model. To some degree, the alternative model is grounded in different social science methodologies. Whereas across-the-board surveys may reveal low scientific literacy, detailed ethnographic studies and in-depth interviews of specific portions of the public (or "publics") reveal a very different picture. The reconstruction model stresses the ways in which the public actively engages and reinterprets scientific knowledge and new technologies (Hess, 1995: chap 6; Wynne 1996). People who do not have advanced degrees in a biomedical field are often able to develop what I call "narrow-band competence" in a specific area of scientific inquiry, such as prostate or breast cancer research, when they are highly motivated to do so. In other words, scientific illiteracy is not an across-the-board phenomenon. Rather than being an amorphous mass of scientific illiterates, the public consists of pockets of strategically grounded literacy and illiteracy. Pockets of the public are capable of becoming quite literate in medical, environmental, and other scientific knowledge when the need arises' (p.229).

The Department of Health, however, has not learned this lesson, as a recent commentary on the MMR controversy indicates:

> *The website where its advice can be found is admirably clear, well set out, and easy to navigate. However, it is striking how many times it uses the word 'expert', as if the use of this mantra will quash any disagreement. The DoH appears not to have noticed that experts are no longer instantly deferred to by the medical profession, let alone the public. The medical profession is struggling to involve patients much more in the decisions concerning their own health and exploring the best ways of achieving this. Lay representation is now familiar on many medical bodies, following the pioneering example of the RCGP* [Royal College of General Practitioners] *many years ago. The DoH may need to recognise that people make decisions for legitimate reasons other than pure science, and that it should include the lay voice, particularly the dissenting voice, when it produces advice in controversial areas.*

> Jewell, 2001, p.876

While the MMR controversy was still raging, a *New Scientist* editorial (16 February 2002) commented:

> *When people have all the facts they can deal with risk. That was the central lesson from the influential inquiry into the Government's handling of the BSE crisis. What will it take to get health officials to learn it?*

Perceptions of risks and benefits

In the MMR example, the issue is in large part one of balancing risks – in this case the perceived risks from the vaccine itself with the risks from the diseases which the vaccine is designed to protect against. In 1998 the Department of Health published *Communicating about Risks to Public Health* (Department of Health, 1998a), which tried to provide guidance to practitioners in handling issues of this kind. As this report makes clear, the perception of the 'expert' and that of the lay person may well be at odds. The development of risk analysis and the various concepts for deciding on appropriate levels of risk have coincided with a growing awareness of the subjectivity of risk perception. Experts and lay people often disagree about the meaning of risk, with the latter at least as concerned with the quality as with the quantifiable and probabilistic impact on their interests. These qualitative factors include two types of subjective risk:

- 'dread risk' involving (in)voluntariness of exposure, potential for catastrophe, the potential overall number of fatalities and so on – for instance, nuclear power, waste disposal and global warming
- 'unknown risk', including characteristics of a hazard which is relatively new, unobservable, potentially delayed and purely hypothetical – for example, embryonic research, cloning and GM foods.

Some of the examples given, such as GM foods, incorporate both types of risk.

The converse of the risk reduction concepts set out in the box opposite would be attempts to communicate the probability of success in certain clinical contexts. In fact, there may be a case for developing means of expressing the uncertainty of success to match ways of communicating the risk of malign consequences. Both positive and adverse effects are highly relevant to medical research, where there may be uncertainty about whether an experimental technique – such as foetal cell transplants – will do harm and the extent to which a complex treatment will provide a benefit.

Sometimes both uncertainties can be present simultaneously, and both will certainly be of concern to patients. Yet it is hard to find substantive discussion of the potential for harm in, for example, the MRC's strategic statements or any other similar document.

The most common conclusion of studies of risk perception is that of amplification: risks often have greater impact on society than statistical calculations of direct harm would suggest they should. In fact, the effect can be more complex than this: even without socio-psychological factors, people may simply misjudge the likelihood of certain events. The classic finding in the literature on bias and risk perception is that people tend to over-estimate the chance of small risks happening, and underestimate the chance of large risks, when compared with the empirical probability of various events actually occurring. Even when information is 'perfect', most people are unable to make sensible estimates of probabilities (Tversky and Kahneman, 1982), and the disjunction between lay public and expert may become still wider.

RISK CONCEPTS

A number of relevant concepts have been developed which are particularly relevant to dealing with the health risks attached to developments inside and outside the health field.

ALARP – As Low As Reasonably Practicable (also **ALARA – As Low As Reasonably Achievable**): This principle is inherent in the Health and Safety at Work Act 1974, regarding the safety of workers and the public in industrial plants. The courts have expressed the view that 'reasonably practicable' was narrower than 'physically possible', thus introducing the possibility that costs of all kinds might be taken into account.

Precautionary Principle: This principle, now in common usage, is colloquially or loosely taken to mean 'if in doubt, don't do it' or 'better to be safe than sorry'. In fact the Phillips Inquiry offered a couple of alternative definitions:

- where the analytical basis for assessment of risk is weak, the lack of full scientific certainty should not be used for postponing cost-effective ['precautionary'] measures particularly where there are threats of serious or irreversible damage
- acting to reduce risk in advance of a complete scientific understanding, by extension of evidence and in the exercise of reasonable foresight.

Both these definitions rather optimistically presume that a time will come where there is 'certainty' or 'complete' understanding. It may be that the precautionary principle is applicable more commonly than this supposes, given our doubts about there ever being 'certainty'.

Proportionality: This European law concept essentially relates to the idea that no more should be done than what is necessary to achieve an objective. In the context, policies to reduce or protect from risk should not devote resources beyond that required to achieve a 'reasonably practicable' level of risk (see above).

NOAEL – No Observable Adverse Effects Level: This is used when licensing medicines or assessing risks in foods from additives or residues. It implies that, perhaps in partial contrast to the precautionary principle, reducing risk beyond that where there is some evidence of harm is not warranted.

Cost/risk-benefit analysis: This concept, familiar to economists, draws attention to the fact that reducing risks will have opportunity costs – perhaps including those risks to other people in other parts of the economy that could be reduced.

Perceptions of conflicts of interest

A further weakening of the 'authority' of science stems from the perception that the apparently disinterested voice of the researcher based in a university or research institute is not in fact disinterested. In December 2001, for example, the *Daily Mail* revealed that the chair of the committee set up to establish the safety of the MMR vaccine had a substantial shareholding in one of its suppliers. As Barlow (1999) has put it: 'The more such conflicts are generally perceived to exist, the less weight will attach to "scientific" opinion and less credence placed on its apparent objectivity.'

The previous chapter remarked on the modification of the incentives facing universities through the development of links with the private sector. The scientific community has itself become sufficiently alarmed about such links to take steps to reduce their significance through the growing requirement for researchers to declare their financial or other interests when, for example, they publish in some learned journals (see, for example, Campbell, 2001).

Diverse priorities

In fact the production of knowledge can never be 'value-free'. When decisions are made to research this rather than that, there is an inherent judgement that one area is more important than another. Even within the public sector, such judgements have been buried within broad statements of 'national priorities', leaving questions about the values to be attached to different kinds of potential benefit to different kinds of patient unasked, still less answered.

In effect, most of the processes described in earlier chapters designed to improve the management of the resources at the disposal of the Department of Health and the NHS rest on the implicit assumption that the issues are essentially technical or expert matters. But, as the attempts to engage consumers in the prioritisation of research funding indicates, this is far from being the case.

Users will attach different values to different projects. They also have different priorities as to what issues projects should address. Many of these areas fall outside what is usually regarded as the domain of science, although not necessarily of systematic study. Examples include the process of care, the experience of disease and of treatment, and the impact of non-financial or physical obstacles on access. In such cases a range of research methods may be applicable, but the data may not be 'hard' and the test of replicability may not apply because each population studied may be unique.

Finally, a more fundamental disjunction: Muir Gray remarks on the popularity of books which do not purport to be based on science, indeed which proclaim the fact they are not as a positive virtue. The existence of such a literature is often dismissed as evidence of the public's irrationality when it comes to health matters. But looked at from a 'market' angle, they could be taken as a sign of deep dissatisfaction with the conventional medical 'product', both in terms of the delivery of care and its content. As a report from the Foundation for Integrated Medicine put it:

> [The] rapid growth in CAM in many western countries suggests a degree of public dissatisfaction with what people see as the limitations of orthodox medicine and concern over the side effect of ever more potent drugs. Biotechnical approaches – pharmaceuticals and surgery – often have a limited amount to offer those with chronic, degenerative or stress-related diseases, mental disorders or addiction.'

Foundation for Integrated Medicine, 1997, p.4

On this view, the development of science-based medicine has overlooked a significant part of the market it might be expected to serve. Naturally enough, those who perceive themselves as neglected turn to other sources of help. A significant proportion of those being treated for cancer by conventional means, for example, also use alternative medicine.

Policy responses

Within the context of the Department of Health/NHS research programme we can find no comprehensive response to the issues raised above. But a recent report from the House of Lords Science and Technology Committee (2000b) focused specifically on the issues raised in the previous section and the Government response to it considered them across Government as a whole (DTI, 2000c).

The House of Lords report identified several areas of concern:

- *The perceived purpose of science is crucial to the public response.*
- *People now question all authority, including scientific authority.*
- *People place more trust in science which is seen as 'independent'.*
- *There is still a culture of governmental and institutional secrecy in the United Kingdom, which invites suspicion.*
- *Some issues currently treated by decision-makers as scientific issues in fact involve many other factors besides science. Framing the problem wrongly by excluding moral, social, ethical and other concerns invites hostility.*
- *What the public finds acceptable often fails to correspond with the objective risks as understood by science. This may relate to the degree to which individuals feel in control and able to make their own choices.*
- *Underlying people's attitudes to science are a variety of values. Bringing these into the debate and reconciling them are challenges for the policy-maker.*

House of Lords, 2000b, p.1

The conclusions and recommendations it made are too numerous to set down here (see the box opposite for a short selection), but their very number indicates the seriousness with which the risk of the public being alienated from science is regarded.

The Government response reported the action being taken already in the areas identified by the Committee across all Government departments. In the field of risk communication it pointed to a wide range of work going on across Government including two Department of Health projects, the first into what people think about health risks and how health risk messages could be improved and the other examining risk literacy. It was also able to point to what the research councils were doing to engage users and others in the process of determining how research resources should be used and what action was being taken to inform and engage the public in scientific developments.

The response also referred to earlier developments in the field of scientific advice in policy making, in particular the Government's commitment to a more open approach.

A code of practice (DTI/OST, 2001a) has been developed (and subsequently revised) bearing on the way that scientific advisory

---

SELECTED RECOMMENDATIONS FROM *SCIENCE AND SOCIETY*

(k) That the Interdepartmental Liaison Group on Risk Assessment should look into current research on how risk information is received by the public (para.4.18).

(l) That direct dialogue with the public should move from being an optional add-on to evidence-based policy making and to the activities of research organisations and learned institutions, and should become a normal and integral part of the process (para.5.48).

(o) That any public dialogue should be conducted in good faith, and that its aims and in particular its role in the policy process should be clear from the start. Those organising public dialogue should see to it that single-issue groups do not monopolise proceedings. The organisers of such events should make every effort to encourage the media to cover the event and to report the outcomes (paras 5.51, 54–55).

(q) That advisory and decision-making bodies in areas involving science should adopt a presumption of openness. This presumption should apply, in particular, to the reasons on which regulatory decisions are made, including all scientific information and advice. The presumption should be overriden only where this can clearly be justified in terms of, for example, genuine commercial confidentiality (para.5.70).

(t) That the scientific merit of particular research grant proposals should continue to be assessed by peer review; but that the Research Councils should do more to involve stakeholders and the public in the wider task of setting the priorities against which particular grants are made, and should seek greater publicity for the process. We suggest that they might seek the considered involvement of Members of Parliament and local authorities, and of other people active in their communities; and that they might hold occasional open forum meetings in different locations (para.5.78).

(House of Lords, 2000b)

---

committees work. It is designed to make the process more open and emphasises the need for departments to:

- think ahead and identify early the issues on which they need scientific advice
- obtain a wide range of advice from the best sources, particularly where there is scientific uncertainty
- publish the scientific advice and all relevant papers.

These points are elaborated in the advice to members and secretariats of the relevant scientific advisory committees who are to regard it as part of their role to:

- consider whether the questions on which the committee offers advice are those which are of interest to the public and other interested parties outside the scientific community
- examine and challenge if necessary the assumptions on which scientific advice is formulated and ask for explanations of any scientific terms and concepts which are not clear
- ensure that the committee has the opportunity to consider contrary scientific views and where appropriate the concerns and values of stakeholders before a decision is taken
- ensure that the committee's advice is comprehensive from the point of view of a lay person.

The Department of Health's *Science and Innovation Strategy* (Department of Health, 2001m) also reports a number of developments within the health field. It notes that the Department is taking the following initiatives:

- a comprehensive internal review of how the Public Health Group in the Department of Health obtains scientific advice
- co-funding with other departments a study to identify good practice in managing scientific advice, which was completed last year. Many Department of Health Advisory Committee members, including lay people, volunteered to take part in this study
- funding research to evaluate different methods of public participation in the advisory process
- participation in cross-Whitehall initiatives on risk assessment and decision making.

And, with regard to communicating with the public:

- new research on expert processes and how we might handle a future BSE-like problem
- funding the Human Genetics Commission to investigate ways of communicating with the public, including open meetings and consultation exercises
- in-house training programmes for staff on managing and communicating risks better.

These are welcome and clearly much-needed developments. They represent the start of what might be a long process of bringing together the ultimate users of that part of the science base which bears on the health economy and those working in it. What is hard to foresee is how, as this dialogue develops, those directing and working within the science base will respond to whatever that dialogue produces.[76] But if this

---

IMPLEMENTATION OF GUIDELINES ON SCIENTIFIC ADVISORY COMMITTEES

The first report on the implementation of these guidelines notes that:

24. One area where this has been particularly significant has been in relation to recent developments in biotechnology. Here the role played by the two new biotechnology commissions, the Human Genetics Commission (HGC) and the Agriculture and Environment Biotechnology Commission (AEBC), has been particularly valuable. These two bodies were set up with a broad membership and a remit to engage the public in debate and to advise Government on the social and ethical implications of new developments in biotechnology. Together with the Food Standards Agency (FSA) they have led the way in developing new and innovative approaches to opening up the scientific advisory process to public scrutiny. It is evident that many of these initiatives are being increasingly adopted across Government for scientific advice in other areas.

The section dealing with the Department of Health reports that:

All key committees advising DH publish their proceedings on the Internet, have lay members and hold open meetings. As a consequence, much of the good practice laid out in the guidance was already in place when they were issued. Improvements have continued since publication of Guidelines 2000 with many DH committees, especially the more newly formed advisory bodies, taking on board many of the recommendations. A review of how Guidelines 2000 have been implemented in DH has highlighted areas where the department is following good practice and also areas where the department could have done better (p.29).

(DTI/OST, 2001b)

---

76. The democratic accountability of science has been the subject of a number of recent studies. See for example Fuller (2000) and Harvey Brown (1998).

dialogue has any substantive content, that ultimately is where it should lead, i.e. some degree of modification to the way in which the resources currently devoted to health-related research are used.

Accountability

We have argued that strain is showing between the worlds of the expert and the scientist on the one hand and of the lay person and ultimate consumer of the output of the health research economy on the other.

First, it seems that the public has grown increasingly aware in practical terms of the underlying philosophical uncertainty of science. Examples of 'failures' such as BSE emerge more clearly as public accountability, information technology, media interest and levels of education open up the previously closed worlds of all kinds of expertise. This is inevitable in modern democracies, and most would argue a good thing too. But it may also reveal a disjunction between the general public and professional researchers in their attitudes to societal change and risk.

As argued above, the average citizen's attitude to risk may well differ sharply from that of the scientific community and policy makers (and the 'average' citizen will not reflect variation in risk perception across the population). This may not simply be a matter of misunderstanding, but one of values and of interests. The individual citizen shares none of the benefits of prestige or financial rewards resulting from scientific innovation, but may bear or fear bearing the costs.

As a result, in a more open and democratic society the issue of how to manage the consumption of knowledge by the whole of society must be tackled. Up to now perhaps too little effort has been devoted to thinking about how we cope with knowledge, and too much to simply going ahead and producing it. The various initiatives mentioned above indicate that this issue has been grasped across Government as a whole, but they represent a beginning rather than a conclusion.

Second, differences of view within science arising in part from differences in method, in part from differences in values and in part from broader cultural factors, argue for a continued emphasis on diversity – for the support of alternative lines of inquiry and the provision of alternative sources of expertise. This point is made in the Code of Practice for scientific advisory committees, but it is not just a question of membership of committees. Some of the measures used to promote the quality of scientific work and its relevance to 'the needs of the NHS' or the 'health of the nation', as well as those designed to foster wealth creation within the public sector, actually work against diversity. As a result dissent may be forced underground – or further underground than it already is. The message to scientific advisory committees that they should be more open should apply to the process of knowledge generation itself.

Third, the process of making the health research economy accountable has only just begun, even within the public sector. This is true at the most basic level: despite the vast amount of information available on the Department's website it is not possible to find any rationale for what is currently being supported or a vision of what kind of health care system the current R&D resources are intended to promote.

The way R&D resources are used has never been examined by any of the normal processes of political accountability – select committee, public accounts committee or professional audit. Instead the unelected and unreconstructed House of Lords has ironically been the main instrument for bringing the issues discussed in this study out into the open.

The Department of Health's emphasis on the three national priorities of cancer, heart disease and mental illness appears to have precluded a wider discussion of the balance of the research programme. We believe that the Department of Health should promote such a discussion. A minimum requirement is a strategic statement of what the current spending is intended to achieve and why the current allocations are as they are. This should comprise the general objectives which it serves and justification of these objectives in the context of the wider health research economy and changes in that economy, the NHS and society at large. It should acknowledge the risks as well as the potential benefits and should make explicit its underlying values, which should, in our view, align with those of the NHS itself.

As for the health research economy as a whole, its accountability can only stem from developments in the relationship between the world of science and society as a whole. As this chapter has shown, the issues are on the table and many measures have been proposed, and some of them implemented, to improve that relationship. Overall, it seems that the time has come to spend more effort on considering what new knowledge we want and how we deal with new knowledge relative to the effort devoted to obtaining it.

In the last analysis, any health care system must command the allegiance of its users and those ultimately financing it. The Government has grasped that issue within the framework of the NHS, with its modernisation programme, its targets and its commitment to extra spending as well as the new initiatives aimed at extending informed consent (see www.doh.gov.uk/informedconsent). But the challenge to clinical authority displayed in the MMR controversy in the first half of 2002 demonstrates the possibility that the NHS as a conventional health care provider may lose that allegiance if it does not recognise the basic shift in the location of knowledge from being the preserve of the professional to a widely available commodity.

Overview

Previous chapters in this study have looked at how the Department of Health has attempted to address deficiencies identified by the House of Lords in 1988 and to deal with issues that have arisen within that broad framework. But the world has moved on since then. A better-informed public is increasingly inclined to question the authority of professionals and scientific experts.

Crises such as that arising from the emergence of nvCJD and disputes such as the one over MMR have led citizens to doubt the conclusions reached by scientists. Greater access to a range of expert opinion enables them to question the decisions of professionals and politicians.

It is not simply a matter of questioning whether scientific knowledge delivers 'the facts'. There are also differences in value and interest. While it may be possible to quantify certain kinds of risk, the resulting conclusions may differ: lay people may not be prepared to accept risks which experts and politicians think are justified. And in the areas where risks are not quantifiable, there is even more scope for disagreement.

Decisions about what areas of research to fund rest on views about priorities. Politicians, professionals, scientists and the public will differ between each other and among themselves about the values that underlie such views. The public is increasingly expecting to have its own views heard when decisions are made.

The Government has begun to recognise the legitimacy of calls for public involvement in science policy making, and to take steps to promote it. So far, however, the steps have been modest and it remains to be seen how the dialogue between research professionals and their ultimate paymasters, the general public, will develop. That it must develop further is essential if the NHS is to retain the allegiance of its users.

Chapter 9

Conclusions and recommendations

The study concludes with an assessment of the many initiatives which have been taken to improve the management of the health research economy and proposes a range of measures to devise a better system.

Conclusions and recommendations

Since the 1998 House of Lords report was published, the machinery for controlling and promoting publicly funded health-related R&D has been substantially altered. The previous chapters have referred to many initiatives which have been taken to improve the way that resources are allocated to health research. In the first part of this chapter we present some broad judgements as to the impact of these measures and in the second we look at some outstanding issues.

What have the new arrangements achieved?

In 1995, the then Secretary of State for Health, Stephen Dorrell, referred to the NHS R&D programme in the following terms:

> a new programme is in place designed to create an effective link between the NHS and the methods and products of science. I believe it has the potential to make the single biggest contribution to patient care in this country.
>
> Department of Health, 1995c, Extract from a speech to the 1st International Conference on the Scientific Basis of Health Services

None of the mass of consultation and other papers emerging from the R&D Directorate has attempted to assess 'progress so far' in realising that potential. The closest to such an assessment is the strategic review of the levy which, although focused on implementation of the Culyer proposals, nevertheless made more general comments about the degree to which the measures taken earlier in the 1990s had been effective. It found that:

> 5. The implementation in 1997 of many of the recommendations of the 1994 report Supporting Research and Development in the NHS (the Culyer Report) initiated a revolution in research management in the NHS. In the few years since the Research & Development programme

has been established every region and major hospital has research & development managed with explicit research and training programmes and plans for future development. Achieving these changes is something with which the NHS can be justifiably proud.

Department of Health, 1999a

Similarly, in 1997 an outside observer, Professor Nick Black, also concluded that considerable progress had been made:

Although it is too soon to establish the value of the R&D program in any rigorous way, some interim assessment is justified, if only to attempt to influence its future direction. The program can be judged a success on several criteria. It has started to redress the balance between basic, clinical, and health services research in terms of funding: raised awareness of and concern for the outcome of health care among clinicians and managers; introduced much greater coherence and logic to research funding decisions; raised the profile and respectability of dissemination and implementation of scientific evidence; mobilized many scientists and clinicians who traditionally were not involved in health care R&D; and funded many research projects and training opportunities. Although none of these can be shown to have benefited the public directly yet, these achievements are necessary stepping stones to that goal.

Black, 1997, p.503

Encouraging though these comments may be, essentially they amount to saying that the management of the NHS R&D programme was moving in the right direction and that its very (well-publicised) existence had helped to encourage a climate favourable to the execution of research and the use of its findings.

That achievement is, nevertheless, a very considerable one. In 1990 Rudolf Klein pointed out that the 'National Health Service ... largely ignores the contribution of the research community' (Klein, 1990). As far as central policy making goes, he would probably repeat that assessment, if in slightly modified form; but as far as the wider NHS goes, he would, if the above assessments are correct, concede that 'the customer' for research is now somewhat better informed than a decade ago.

The main evidence for that lies not so much within the R&D programme itself, as in the rapid development during the 1990s of new journals such as *Bandolier* and new activities such as the Cochrane collaborations. These are based on the systematic use of the existing knowledge base and reflect a greater appetite for using the results of research throughout the NHS.

It is harder to find evidence, however, that the full range of issues raised in the 1988 House of Lords report have been fully addressed – not to mention those considered in Chapter 8. In particular, although progress has been made in particular areas, the record does not suggest that overall there is now a much closer fit between the R&D that is carried out within the Department of Health's field of responsibility and 'the needs of the NHS'. The analysis commissioned internally – the strategic review of the levy – revealed substantial shortfalls in achievement. Our own analysis has revealed serious weaknesses in all the areas we have considered. We briefly rehearse them below before drawing out some general conclusions.

Finance

The system by which resources are allocated to R&D within the Department of Health and the NHS rests on inadequate foundations. As the experience of the House of Lords Science and Technology Committee demonstrates, how the resources currently being devoted to R&D are actually used within the NHS remains uncertain as to the topics they cover and the quality of the work they produce. Reforms are under way which will produce greater clarity. However, as official papers make clear, it will be some time before these will be far enough advanced to underpin a principled reallocation of resources beyond the modest programmes already supported by central funding in the national priority areas and the centrally run programmes themselves.

The relationship between the form of funding and the current failures of the supply side of the health research economy remain to be substantively addressed. The scope for redirecting research is limited by weaknesses on the supply side. While these weaknesses arise from many factors, one is the way that finance is allocated. The timescale for building up an effective research capacity in this area (and others) is much longer than that governing the allocation of finance. While the

Director of R&D should soon be able to form a clearer view of the current balance of spending, the reforms in progress are not guided by an explicit vision of what the provider side should consist of and what its weaknesses currently are.

The balance of spending

As we have noted, the composition of the then pattern of spending was one of the key features singled out for criticism in the House of Lords 1988 report. Whether any or all of these claims were justified and whether or not there has been an effective response, it is impossible to say. But the central criticism made by the 1988 Committee that the Department and the NHS were not effective at generating ideas as to their research needs, has been addressed, at least in part. The process described in Chapter 3 has led to a series of documents, each setting out substantial research agenda for particular subject areas and, to a modest extent, new programmes have resulted.

However, it is also clear that these programmes of work have not been adequate. The latest attempts to define broad areas of work for the three main priority areas – within the Cancer Plan and the national service frameworks for mental illness and heart disease – indicate that even the focused reviews have not led to programmes of work which are based on a strategic view of each of these priority areas.

Furthermore the Department of Health has still not produced a principled approach to the allocation of research monies. It continues to focus on 'national priorities', but it has defined these in terms of diseases, not in terms of what Government policy towards the NHS is trying to achieve. Moreover, by focusing on three conditions, albeit major ones, it has implicitly downplayed other important areas such as stroke or diabetes, not to mention diseases affecting small groups of people for whom an equity case can be made.

Equally significant, there is no sign that 'the needs of the NHS' have been adequately assessed. This is just not a matter of individual topics, professions or diseases, but rather what an organisation such as the NHS requires if it is to improve performance. There is almost no sign of a recognition of the need to shift the emphasis in research away from the search for exact answers to precise questions towards the derivation of knowledge and information which can be helpful, even if not conclusive, in dealing with broad-ranging questions such as what 'the hospital of the future' should look like or meeting day-to-day needs of service redesign at local level. As the figures presented in Chapter 1 showed, the share of research spending within the NHS which the NHS instigates is modest and, within that, only a fraction is likely to be devoted to questions of this sort.

Finally, our own analysis of gaps, on both the payer and the provider side of the health research economy, defined in terms of topics, disciplines or fields suggests that the central issue of what the role of publicly financed research should be has not been directly addressed. Determining what this should be must start, given the nature of the health research economy, with an assessment of the role of the private sector and the scope for influencing what it does in the direction of ends determined by health policy objectives rather than wealth creation. Recent official papers conflate these two objectives and hence implicitly assume that what is good for 'Big Pharm' is also good for the NHS.

Supply

The supply side of the health research economy remains poorly developed. The Department has taken initiatives such as those represented in the workforce capacity development project which recognise some of the existing weaknesses. However, these look modest in scale set against the deep-rooted obstacles identified in Chapter 5.

Furthermore, the challenges of interdisciplinary, long-term and innovatory research have yet to be met. A number of ideas have emerged – the laboratory, the system, the local health economy – but so far they have not received sufficient attention as the basis for thinking about 'the needs of the NHS' and the best way of meeting them. As things currently stand, some kinds of research are almost impossible to envisage as practical possibilities because the institutions capable of executing them do not exist.

Interfaces

There have been many initiatives designed to promote the collective working of the health research economy, particularly those parts financed from public funds. How effective these have been is impossible to tell. It is clear, however, that many issues remain unresolved or indeed unrecognised. Evidence such as that from the Nuffield studies suggests the interfaces between the NHS and the universities remain unsatisfactory, as does evidence presented to the House of Commons Science and Technology Committee in relation to cancer research in particular.

The cancer example suggests that the Department of Health does not yet have the capacity to take a strategic view of any one area or to define its role in relation to the other actors. More generally, it has not set out a strategy for its contribution to the health research economy as a whole, based on a considered view of the scale and nature of the contributions of its various elements. While it has begun to put in place the basis for a partnership with the private sector, this is not founded on a systematic analysis of the weaknesses of the overall health research economy from the viewpoint of the NHS.

Overall

The summary judgements set out above may seem harsh,[77] but they can nearly all be traced to official documents. From the Culyer report through the review of the levy to the consultation papers and other documents appearing during 2000 and the follow-up papers in 2001, it is clear that a lot remains to be done before the 1988 criticisms can be fully dealt with. Essentially all these documents represent work in progress.

Thus the most favourable overall conclusion to be drawn as to the effectiveness of Department of Health policy towards publicly funded health-related R&D might be that the process of reforming the finance and management of the NHS R&D programme is still under way and some key elements have yet to appear, but that the overall direction is right. But is it?

Our analysis suggests that, despite the vast effort which has been devoted to improving the way resources are used within the health research economy since 1988, a number of important issues continue to be systematically ignored.

Chapter 8 argued that since 1988 'the game has moved on'. The key change since 1988 lies in how 'the knowledge base of the NHS' is envisaged. The 1988 report correctly identified a series of important

---

77. Mark Baker in the final chapter of Baker and Kirk (1998) also comes to a critical conclusion on the R&D programme as a whole. See in particular pp.158–60.

weaknesses, but its mental frame of reference reflected the 'old-style' professional roles rather than the 'new-style' roles which are beginning to emerge. The new mental frame of reference involves not only a recognition of a shift in clinical relationships, but also a change in the understanding of what counts as knowledge and how it should be obtained. In other words, the nature of the 'best possible contribution' to be made by research to the NHS has changed and is changing further.

There is no mechanistic way of defining what the 'best possible' collection of projects actually is. In the absence of such a methodology, the criteria relevant to judging whether the programme is achieving the 'best possible' disposition must necessarily be of a rather general nature, bearing on the way that the health research economy is structured rather than the selection of particular research areas. Our analysis suggests the following broad criteria:

- All areas of potential research must have a chance of inclusion – the existing health research economy is diverse, but not diverse enough.
- Different views as to the value of different uses of research monies should be heard. The institutional diversity of the health research economy should not be suppressed by uniformity of view as to what counts as valid research nor, more fundamentally, as to what areas are worth investigating.
- The process of determining the balance of research between broad areas and within them should be transparent and the criteria used to determinate how resources are allocated should be explicit.
- The suppliers of research must not dominate in determining the composition of the programme, but they should retain a voice. Clearly in some areas they are best placed to propose what work should be done and what new areas are worth investigating. This is particularly true in those areas of research which are not closely linked to a particular problem or disease.
- The basis for whatever judgements are made as to the allocation of research resources within the NHS R&D programme should be explicit and the allocation between competing uses justified with reference to those criteria. More generally, means should be found for bringing a greater degree of accountability into research supported by the Department of Health/NHS – but not at the price of infringing the principles set out above. That is to say there should be scope in all the main parts of the health research economy for a degree of 'free-wheeling' away from detailed contractual arrangements.

- The way that the UK disposes of its research resources should be determined in part by reference to the world health research economy. (We have not argued this point in this study, but it seems self-evident, given the relative scale of the UK and the world health research economy.)

As we have seen, whether these requirements are met depends as much on the supply of research as on the demand for it. Both sides of the health research economy have to function properly, but the evidence we have briefly summarised above suggests that neither does. In particular:

- The proper division of roles between public and private sectors remains to be clarified.
- There remains no clear sense of how research funding within the NHS should be directed and managed even in those areas defined as national priorities, still less in those which (according to our analysis and that of others) suffer from neglect.
- It is not clear whose job it now is to think about the health research economy as a whole and its relationship with the public.

In the next part we stand back from the details of policy development and take each of these areas. We consider some of the fundamental questions which it would seem from the policy record have so far been given insufficient attention.

What next? Some recommendations

Funding a diversity of research

- An organisation should be created to act as budget-holder with the task of taking systematic stock of the whole field of health research and targeting funds on areas where a case can be made for 'neglect'.
- An important role of the budget-holder would be to protect and promote diversity in the health research economy.
- This organisation should have a limited life span.

Our first proposal concerns the proper funding structure within the public sector. The 1988 report argued that the right place to locate control of the overall budget was outside the Department of Health, while the

Government argued for a locus within the Department. Both were agreed that there should be one central focus. Our analysis casts some doubt on this.

The vision implicit in the measures being taken to manage the existing programme better is that a single considered view (to which, it has to be recognised, a wider range of views contribute than would have been the case in the 1980s) is the most effective way of determining what research should be carried out in each field. The establishment of a National Cancer Institute is the latest manifestation of that approach.

Clearly there are strong arguments for some organisation, actual or virtual, taking an overview of a broad field such as cancer. But there is also a risk that such an approach will lead to the kind of market failure which arises from the socialisation of science.[78] In cancer and many other areas there are deep-seated controversies, within medical research and the wider scientific community, as well as between that community and others, about the most fruitful areas to which research should be directed (see, for example, Hess, 1997; Epstein, 1998; Baum, 2002).

Furthermore, we have noted the widespread concern in the wider scientific community (Campbell, 2001) about the biases being introduced into the way science operates and the 'corruption' of the main centres for independent research – the universities. The arguments set out in Chapter 6 suggested that encouraging academics and their institutions to develop knowledge and commercial products in neglected areas may at the same time undermine their independence, as well as reducing the overall efficiency of the health research economy through the privatisation of knowledge.

Accordingly we believe that a substantial stream of public funding should be reserved for the support of areas which the existing players are reluctant to support. The not-for-profit sector currently *de facto* acts like this, but it too has its 'market failures' and biases. Although some areas of work such as cancer are well endowed, others are not, and even within cancer some areas find it hard to stake a claim to funding.

In proposing this, we take it as read that diversity of both payers and providers is desirable in research for precisely the same reasons it is

---

78. This has been the main criticism levied at the US National Cancer Institute, by Epstein (1998), for example.

generally desirable for other goods and services. A system dominated by the State, the private sector or one profession – or even one sector of one profession – would entail the risk that only one set or only a limited set of views were heard as to what 'the needs of the NHS' are and how they should be met.[79]

Such diversity may have to be protected and promoted, even possibly within the Department of Health/NHS programme, through the creation of an organisation to act as budget-holder. The budget-holder would be tasked with taking systematic stock of the whole field and, against that background, target funds on areas where a case can be made for 'neglect'. In some areas of work its role might be to convince existing providers of the merits of changing their current portfolio; in others its role would be to commission work in its own right, particularly where there is no established provider. No existing organisation is suited for this task since all are identified with parts of the system; some new vehicle would have to be devised. Given the spirit of this recommendation, any such organisation should itself only have a finite life say of ten years to reduce the risks of capture by one 'vested' interest or another.[80, 81]

---

79. Hardy (2001) makes the point that in a climate in which 'what matters is what works': 'Policy research becomes more about how to solve the problem than what the problem might be ... in such a world, radical thought becomes less important.' In other words, new and divergent thinking becomes virtually impossible to fund. In his words, 'you cannot get money for a number of absolutely key issues'. His remarks are directed not just at health, but at the policy world more generally.

80. McLachlan suggested a long time ago that 'independent judgement is desirable ... for the assessment of the conclusions likely to be drawn from the development of information technology'. He argued that 'the ethos of such a body requires that it should be multi-disciplined and insulated from the direct influence of those concerned with the formation of public policy and its execution' (McLachlan, 1990, p.204).

81. Cohen (1981) remarked that 'the scale and scope of the Department's policy concerned, and of research which underpins it, means that the construction of some grand design in which all the elements are in place is unlikely to succeed.'

A shift of resources towards the operation of the NHS

Substantially more resources should be allocated to research in those areas where clinical, managerial and organisational issues intersect. The following measures should be taken to achieve this:

- Existing regulators should be enabled to exploit more fully the data they collect and to finance supporting studies.
- There should be much larger spending on researching how the NHS is used, on mechanisms of service delivery and on innovations in service delivery.
- New research techniques should be developed to deal with complexity.
- A small number of new research institutions should be established to conduct large-scale, system-wide studies.

Our second proposal is targeted at the main gap identified in 1988 and reaffirmed by our own analysis, i.e. the operation of the NHS. In our view, the response so far has been too little and too late, given the vast number of unknowns involved in the implementation of the NHS Plan. With the massive injection of funds which the Government is now providing, however, the basic need to ensure they are well used is as great as ever. Indeed, the Government has recognised this through the vast range of regulators it has now established – the Commission for Health Improvement, the Modernisation Agency, the National Patient Safety Agency and so on.

In the course of their work, these new regulators and the existing ones, generate a vast amount of information about how the service works and where it does not work well. They do not, however, have the resources to exploit that information in full or to carry out or finance supporting studies designed to complement it. In other words, regulators need their own knowledge base. Among other things, this means that they should have the capacity to exploit in academic ways the data they and only they can collect and to distil from the knowledge provided by the health research economy what they require to carry out their own work.

We believe that there should be a systematic shift of resources towards the delivery end of the research spectrum – to those areas where clinical, managerial and organisational issues intersect. This could involve the following:

- much larger spending on gaining knowledge of how the NHS is used and what happens to the patients within it, e.g. the flow of patients through a cancer care system, developing the cancer registry system and copying its relevant features to other conditions
- the development of new analytic and research techniques to deal with complexity and the need to cope with the interaction of a large number of interventions and external factors
- much larger spending on innovation in service delivery, including development of contracts with the private sector to define new ways of designing health care facilities and delivering the services within them
- major experiments taking in systems of care, to allow comparisons across the NHS of alternative delivery mechanisms
- the development of a small number of new research institutions capable of mounting large-scale system-wide studies on a much bigger scale than any currently envisaged.

Defining the State's role in relation to the private sector

A task force should be set up with members from the public sector, the pharmaceutical industry and charitable funders to consider private–public relationships from a health viewpoint. It should consider how new regulations and/or financial incentives could overcome market failures which lead to gaps in health research.

The third proposal concerns the relationship between the role of the State and the role of the private sector. Although much has been written about this relationship in specific terms, and particularly the price regulation of pharmaceuticals, the R&D programme does not appear to have reached an overarching view of the particular advantages which the State can bring to bear.

Chapter 6 concluded that, despite the close relationship between Government and industry, there has been no effective discussion of public and private roles across *all* the areas where those roles should be defined. The precise terms of the public–private partnership between the

Department of Health and the pharmaceutical industry have only just been resolved at the most elementary level, i.e. in the areas of cost sharing, facility pricing and data availability.

Similarly, there has been no effective debate as to whether or not there should be a proactive public role in drugs and devices in response to market failure in areas such as orphan drugs or alternative medicines. The recently announced partnership agreement between the Department of Health and the pharmaceutical industry partially recognises the need for a proactive role, but it applies to only one part, albeit an important one, of the spectrum of actual and possible public–private relationships.

Earlier chapters set out how the 'free market' for research fails. Chapter 2 reviewed the roles of the main players in the health research economy and set out in some detail where these failures may occur: Chapter 6 gave some examples. What is now needed is a pharmaceutical industry/charitable funder/Government task force which considers public–private relationships from the health viewpoint. This would cover the gaps we and others have identified and consider ways in which new forms of regulation or financial incentives might overcome some of these failures. Where this is not feasible or not cost-effective, then new forms of public action may be required, probably, though not necessarily, in partnership with the private sector.

Transparency and communication

- Politicians and scientific experts should be prepared to be more honest about the limits of knowledge, giving advice which acknowledges uncertainties, disagreements and risks.
- The views of experts should be given due weight, but they should be subordinated to the will of the people and their representatives.
- More effort should be devoted to thinking about how we cope with the knowledge generated by the health research economy.

Finally, the health research economy's relationship with the public. Chapter 8 reviewed the ways in which professional (and State) authority was being undermined. We conclude with a number of thoughts about the general direction in which future policy should lead.

It seems most important to develop more brutal honesty about the limits of science and the nature and existence of risks, particularly by avoiding notions of 'absolute certainty' or 'complete safety'. This applies to all science, of course, and not just the medical and health field. Such a development might involve a move from the expert advisory committee providing dispassionate and 'private' advice to the politician, to a more open system of advice-giving, where experts are free to disagree with one another, and the politicians are given the task of adjudicating between them. The measures described in Chapter 8 are a step in this direction. So too are the steps being taken by NICE to engage both experts and non-experts in their deliberations (see www.nice.org.uk).

The public at large is now well aware that experts disagree, and to pretend that there is an unequivocally 'right' answer in these circumstances will simply serve to bring the whole of public decision making further into disrepute. Open acknowledgement that the final decision rests on what is essentially a judgement about evidence, rather than absolute truth, should lead to a more mature public debate about scientific advance.

The politicians for their part should show a greater readiness either to resist or to go further than scientific advice in their role as public representatives, even when this 'expert' advice appears to hold unanimous support in professional circles. This reflects the fact, discussed in Chapter 8, that the lay perception of risk may differ in a very real way from that held by experts whose professional life is devoted to such matters.

In other cases, where probabilities are harder to define, the response to potential hazards can differ markedly between a scientist whose career will benefit from technical advance, and the ordinary citizen who simply has to live with the uncertainty that that advance brings in its wake. Genetic modification probably provides the clearest example of such a situation, but in smaller ways it applies to many new medical treatments and therapies where long-term effects are unknown, such as hormone replacement therapy. It is impossible to prove that something cannot happen: 'proof' only occurs when a hypothesis that a disastrous event cannot happen is itself disproved – obviously requiring the event itself to take place! Thus politicians and individuals have to make judgements beyond the realms of scientific 'certainty'.

This leaves us with a puzzle about the role of the 'expert'. On the one hand, experts do have more knowledge than lay people, simply by virtue of being paid to devote time and effort to thinking about them – it would be rather disconcerting if they did not. But, equally, experts disagree among themselves and, for the reasons alluded to earlier in this study, we cannot and must not accept what they say without question.

So how can we balance these observations? The answer does not present itself easily. But it seems clear that we will in the future need to perceive the expert as someone whose voice may carry special weight but not the final answer, and whose influence should perhaps be greater than the views of ordinary members of the public but not override them. Not to admit a special position for those who devote themselves to studying an issue is perverse. But, as the developments in the role and conduct of scientific advisory committees acknowledges, the realm of their influence should be carefully constrained, the content of their advice open to scrutiny, and ultimately their role firmly subordinated to the will of the people and their representatives.

All this leads to a final recommendation. The issue of how to manage the consumption of knowledge by the *whole* of society has been given too low a priority up to now. As we suggested in the previous chapter, perhaps too little effort is devoted to thinking about how we cope with knowledge, and too much with simply going ahead and producing it. A new research agenda emerges: that of learning how to communicate and share the very process of learning itself.

Bibliography

Abraham J (1996). *Science, politics and the pharmaceutical industry: Controversy and bias in drug regulation*. London: UCL Press.

Abraham J, Lewis G (2001). Secrecy and transparency of medicines licensing in the EU. *Lancet*; 352: 480–82.

Advisory Committee on Dangerous Pathogens (1996). *Microbiological risk assessment: An interim report*. London: HMSO.

Anderson J, Fears R, editors (1997). *Hard choices: Shaping public science policy for the new millennium*. Oxted: ScienceBridge.

Anderson J, Fears R, editors (1996). *Sustaining the strength of the UK in healthcare and life sciences R&D: Competition, cooperation and cultural change*. Oxted: ScienceBridge.

Arnold E, Morrow S, Thuriaux B, Martin B (1999). *Implementing the Culyer reforms in North Thames: Final report*. Science and Technology Policy Research, Technopolis.

ARMS (2001). *Careers in research: Research proposals of the Committee of the Association of Researchers in Medicine and Science*. Manchester: University of Manchester. Accessed at www.hop.man.as.uk/arms/PROPOSAL

Austoker J (1988). *A history of the Imperial Cancer Research Fund 1902–1986*. Oxford: Oxford University Press.

Bagshawe K D, chair (1984). *Acute services for cancer: Report of a working group*. London: Standing Medical Advisory Committee.

Baker M (2001). NHS R&D: future prospects. In: Baker M, Kirk S, editors. *Research and development for the NHS: Evidence, evaluation and effectiveness*. 2nd ed. Oxford: Radcliffe Medical Press, 58–60.

Baker M, Kirk S, editors (2001). *Research and development for the NHS: Evidence, evaluation and effectiveness*. 2nd ed. Oxford: Radcliffe Medical Press.

Barlow T (2001). When the devil invites you to dine. *Weekend Financial Times* 26/27 May: II.

Barlow T (1999). Science plc. *Prospect* August/September: 36.

Barr N (1998). *The economics of the welfare state*. Oxford: Oxford University Press.

Bauer H H (2001). *Science or pseudoscience: Magnetic healing, psychic phenomena, and other heterodoxies*. Urbana and Chicago: University of Illinois Press.

Baum M (2002). A new strategy for cancer. *Prospect* February: 44–48.

BBC News (2001). Stroke research warning. *BBC News online* 18 May.

Berwick D (2002). Commentary: same price, better care. *BMJ*; 324: 142–43

Black N (1997). A national strategy for research and development: Lessons from England. *Annual Review of Public Health*; 18: 485–505.

Briggs A, Shelley J H, editors (1986). *Science, medicine and the community: The last hundred years.* Proceedings of the Fifth Boehringer Ingelheim Symposium held at Kronberg, Taunus 8–11 May 1985. Amsterdam: Excerpta Medica.

Bunker J, Nuffield Trust (2001). *Medicine matters for all: Measuring the benefits of medical care, a healthy lifestyle, and a just social environment.* London: The Stationery Office.

Buxton M, Hanney S (1998). Evaluating the NHS research and development programme: Will the programme give value for money? *Journal of the Royal Society of Medicine*; 91 (Suppl.35): 2–7b.

Buxton M, Hanney S (1996). How can payback from health services research be assessed? *Journal of Health Services Research and Policy*; 1(1): 35–43c.

Buxton M, Hanney S (1994). *Assessing payback from Department of Health research and development: Preliminary report. Vol. 1: The main report.* Uxbridge: Brunel University.

Cabinet Office (2000). *The Government response to the House of Lords Select Committee on Science and Technology Third Report, Science and Society.* Cm 4875. London: The Stationery Office.

Cabinet Office, Office of Public Service and Science, Office of Science and Technology (1993). *A report on medical research and health.* London: HMSO.

Cabinet Office (1972). *Framework for Government research and development.* Cm 5046. London: HMSO.

Cabinet Office Advisory Council on Science and Technology (1993). *A report on medical research and health.* London: HMSO.

Callahan D (1999). *False hopes: Overcoming the obstacles to a sustainable, affordable medicine.* New Brunswick, NJ: Rutgers University Press.

Calman K, Hine D, chairs (1995). *A policy framework for commissioning cancer services: A report by the Expert Advisory Group on Cancer to the Chief Medical Officers of England and Wales. Guidance for purchasers and providers of cancer services.* London: Department of Health.

Campbell P (2001). Declaration of financial interests. *Nature*; 412: 751.

Central Health Services Council (1971). *Report of the Central Health Services Council for the year ended 31st December, 1970, preceded by a statement made by the Secretary of State for Social Services and the Secretary of State for Wales.* London: HMSO.

Centre for Policy in Nursing Research, Royal College of Nursing, Research Forum for Allied Health Professionals, Association of Commonwealth Universities (2001). *Promoting research in nursing and the allied health professions.* Research Report 01/64. Higher Education Funding Council for England.

Cohen R (1981). The DHSS and the MRC: the first Chief Scientist looks back. In: McLachlan G, editor. *Matters of moment: Management, inner cities, maternity, collaboration.* Oxford: Oxford University Press for the Nuffield Provincial Hospitals Trust; 1–24.

Coleman V (1977). *Paper doctors: A critical assessment of medical research.* London: Maurice Temple Smith Ltd.

Committee on NIH Research Priority-Setting Process (1998). *Scientific opportunities and public needs: Improving priority setting and public input at the National Institutes of Health.* Washington DC: National Academy Press.

Costa D L (2000). *Long-term declines in disability among older men: Medical care, public health, and occupational change.* Working Paper 7605. Cambridge, Mass: National Bureau of Economic Research.

Cowper A (2002). NICE: Still advancing the excellence curve. *British Journal of Health Care Management*; 8: 92–95.

Culyer A J (1994a), chair. *Supporting research and development in the NHS.* Report of the Department of Health Research and Development Task Force. London: HMSO.

Culyer A (1994b). *Funding Research in the NHS.* York: University of York.

Culyer A (1998). *Economics and public policy – NHS research and development as a public good.* Discussion Paper 163. York: University of York.

Dalziel M (2000). *Using research to improve health care services.* Available from www.sdo.lshtm.ac.uk.

Davis P, editor (1996). *Contested ground: Public purpose and private interest in the regulation of prescription drugs.* Oxford: Oxford University Press.

Dawson G *et al* (1998). *Mapping the landscape.* London: Wellcome Trust.

DeAngelis C D (2000). Conflict of interest and the public trust. *JAMA*; 284: 2237–38.

Department of Health (2002a). *Government response to Bristol Royal Infirmary report.* PR 2002/0030. London: Department of Health.

Department of Health (2002b). *Partnership will enable joint funding of clinical research.* PR 2002/0155. London: Department of Health.

Department of Health (2002c). *NHS research capacity development.* doh.gov.uk/research/rd3/workforcecapacity.htm.

Department of Health (2001a). *Pharmaceutical Industry Competitiveness Taskforce report.* London: Department of Health.

Department of Health (2001b). *Lord Hunt announces new health technology device research programme.* PR 2001/0466. London: Department of Health.

Department of Health (2001c). *A research and development strategy for public health.* London: Department of Health.

Department of Health (2001d). *Extra resources for local health services. Research and development budget to rise 6.6%.* PR 2001/0069. London: Department of Health.

Department of Health (2001e). *R&D research governance framework for health and social care.* London: The Stationery Office.

Department of Health (2001f). *NHS priorities and needs R&D funding: A position paper.* London: The Stationery Office.

Department of Health (2001g). *National service framework – for older people.* London: The Stationery Office.

Department of Health (2001h). *Lord Hunt announces £8 million for research into ageing and services for older people.* PR 2001/0536. London: Department of Health.

Department of Health (2001i). *NHS announces crucial investment in new research: Primary care development awards exceed £2.5 million in third year.* London: Department of Health.

Department of Health (2001j). *Lord Hunt announces new health technology device research programme.* London: Department of Health.

Department of Health (2001k). *The expert patient.* London: The Stationery Office.

Department of Health (2001l). *Research and development for a first class service: Next steps.* London: Department of Health.

Department of Health (2001m). *Science and innovation strategy.* London: Department of Health.

Department of Health (2001n). *R&D information for health and social care.* Downloadable from www.doh.gov.uk.

Department of Health (2000a). *Towards a strategy for nursing research and development: Proposals for action.* London: Department of Health.

Department of Health (2000b). *Research and development for a first class service.* London: Department of Health.

Department of Health (2000c). *Government response to the sixth report of the House of Commons Science and Technology Committee: Session 1999/2000. Cancer research – A fresh look.* London: The Stationery Office.

Department of Health (2000d). *PPRS – Fourth report to Parliament.* London: The Stationery Office.

Department of Health. *NHS R&D funding. Consultation paper: NHS priorities and needs R&D funding.* London: Department of Health, 2000e.

Department of Health. *Pharmacy Plan.* London: The Stationery Office, 2000f.

Department of Health. *NHS R&D funding. Consultation paper: NHS support for science.* London: The Stationery Office, 2000g.

Department of Health (2000h). *£1m cash boost for prostate cancer research. New action plan being developed to improve treatment and care.* PR 2000/0127. London: Department of Health.

Department of Health (2001i). *The NHS Cancer Plan: A plan for investment; a plan for reform.* Leeds: Department of Health.

Department of Health (2000j). *The NHS Plan: A plan for investment; a plan for reform.* Cm 4818-I. London: The Stationery Office.

Department of Health (2000k). *New EC Regulation offers fresh incentives for the production of orphan drugs.* PR 2000/0510. London: Department of Health.

Department of Health (1999a). *Strategic review of the NHS R&D levy: Final report.* London: Department of Health.

Department of Health (1999b). *Saving lives: our healthier nation.* London: The Stationery Office.

Department of Health (1999c). *Topic working group report, Ageing and age-associated disease and disability.* London: Department of Health.

Department of Health (1999d). *Topic working group report, Strategic priorities in cancer research and development.* London: Department of Health.

Department of Health (1999e). *Topic working group report, NHS R&D strategic review: Coronary heart disease and stroke.* London: Department of Health.

Department of Health (1999f). *Topic working group report, Mental health topic working group, final report.* London: Department of Health.

Department of Health (1999g). *Topic working group report, NHS R&D strategic review: Primary care.* London: Department of Health.

Department of Health (1999h). *Topic working group report, Strategic review of research priorities for accidental injury.* London: Department of Health.

Department of Health (1999i). *Making a difference: Strengthening the nursing, midwifery and health visiting contribution to health and healthcare.* London: Department of Health.

Department of Health (1998a). *Communicating about risks to public health: Pointers to good practice.* London: The Stationery Office.

Department of Health (1998b). *Developing human resources for health-related R&D: Next steps. Report of the R&D Workforce Capacity Development Group.* London: Department of Health.

Department of Health (1998c). *Research and Development*, Issue 6, London: Department of Health.

Department of Health (1997a). *Dobson to appoint nursing professor to boost nursing research.* PR 97/251. London: Department of Health, 29 September.

Department of Health (1997b). *Research and development funding boosted for new strategy to improve patient care.* PR 97/361. London: Department of Health, 27 November.

Department of Health (1997c). *Policy research programme 1997.* London: HMSO.

Department of Health (1997d). *Strategic framework for the use of the NHS R&D levy.* London: HMSO.

Department of Health (1997e). *R&D support funding for NHS providers.* London: Department of Health.

Department of Health (1996a). *Research capacity strategy for the Department of Health and the NHS: A first statement.* London: HMSO.

Department of Health (1996b). *Primary care: Delivering the future.* London: HMSO.

Department of Health (1995a). *Consumer research in the NHS: Consumer issues within the NHS.* London: HMSO.

Department of Health (1995b). *Consumers and research in the NHS: Involving consumers in local health care.* London: HMSO.

Department of Health (1995c). *NHS research & development programme poised to revolutionise patient care in the next century – Stephen Dorrell.* PR 95/460. London: Department of Health.

Department of Health (1995d). *Supporting research and development in the NHS. A declaration of NHS activity and costs associated with research and development: Initial guidance.* London: Department of Health.

Department of Health (1995e). *Priorities in medical research: The Government response.* London: HMSO.

Department of Health (1995f). *R&D briefing pack 1995.* London: HMSO.

Department of Health (1995g). *Medical research and the NHS reforms: Government response to the third report on the House of Lords Select Committee on Science and Technology: 1994–95 session.* London: HMSO.

Department of Health (1995h). *NHS R&D programme poised to revolutionise patient care in the next century.* PR 95/440. London: Department of Health.

Department of Health (1995i). *The nursing and therapy professions' contribution to health services research and development. Report of a conference held on 12 May 1994.* London: HMSO.

Department of Health (1994a). *R&D priorities in relation to the interface between primary and secondary care.* London: HMSO.

Department of Health (1994b). *R&D priorities in cancer: Report to the NHS Central Research and Development Committee.* London: Department of Health.

Department of Health (1993a). *Report of the Taskforce on the Strategy for Research in Nursing, Midwifery and Health Visiting.* London: HMSO.

Department of Health (1993b). *Research for Health.* London: Department of Health.

Department of Health (1992). *Review of the role of DH-funded research units: Strategies for long-term funding of research and development.* London: Department of Health.

Department of Health (1991a). *Research for health: A research and development strategy for the NHS.* London: HMSO.

Department of Health (1991b). *The health of the nation: A consultative document for health in England presented to Parliament by the Secretary of State for Health, June 1991.* London: HMSO.

Department of Health (1990). *Department of Health yearbook of research and development 1990.* London: HMSO.

Department of Health (1989). *Priorities in medical research: Government response to the third report of the House of Lords Select Committee on Science and Technology: 1987–88 session.* London: HMSO.

Department of Health/HEFCE (2000). *Statement of strategic alliance on research and development for health and social care.* London: The Stationery Office.

Department of Health/Pharmaceutical Industry Competitiveness Task Force (2002). *Clinical research report.* London: Department of Health.

Department of Health and Social Security (1981). *Growing older.* Cmnd. 8173. London: HMSO.

Dinsmore J (2001). Poor catch from fishing in our gene pool. *Medicine Today*; 1: 6–7.

Doern GB, Reed T, editors (2000). *Risky business: Canada's changing science-based policy and regulatory regime.* Toronto: University of Toronto Press Inc.

Drews J (1999). *In quest of tomorrow's medicines.* New York: Springer.

DTI (2002). *Realising our potential.* London: The Stationery Office.

DTI (2001a). *Hewitt announces outcome of research council review.* PR OP/2001/683. London: Department of Trade and Industry.

DTI (2001b). *New code to help public confidence in science.* PR P/2001/727. London: Department of Trade and Industry.

DTI (2001c). *Byers announces £40m to turn bright ideas into business successes.* PR P/2001/224. London: Department of Trade and Industry.

DTI (2001d). *Universities to be drivers of growth.* PR P/2001/229. London: Department of Trade and Industry.

DTI (2000a). *£129 million cash boost for UK university research.* PR 2000/241. London: Department of Trade and Industry.

DTI (2000b). *Excellence and opportunity: A science and innovation policy for the 21st century.* London: The Stationery Office.

DTI (2000c). *Government response to the House of Lords Select Committee on Science and Technology third report: Science and society.* London: The Stationery Office.

DTI (2000d). *Hearts and minds benefit from £71m science boost.* Press Release. London: Department of Trade and Industry, 9 March.

DTI/OST (2001a). *Code of practice for scientific advisory committees.* London: Department of Trade and Industry.

DTI/OST (2001b). *Scientific advice and policy making: Implementation of guidelines 2000. Report by the Chief Scientific Adviser, Professor David King.* London: Department of Trade and Industry.

DTI/OST (2001c). *Foresight. Health care 2020.* London: The Stationery Office.

DTI/OST (1995). *Technology progress through partnership 4: Health and life science.* London: HMSO.

DTI/OST (1993). *Medical research and health.* London: HMSO.

DTI/OST/Wellcome Trust (2000). *Science and the public: A review of science communication and public attitudes to science in Britain.* London: DTI.

Easmon C (1998). *The universities and the NHS – Managing the markets.* 1997/98 NHS Handbook; 243–51.

Edwards A, Elwyn G (2001). Understanding risk and lessons for clinical risk communication about treatment preferences. *Quality in Health Care*; 10(Suppl.I): i9–i13.

Enserink M (2001). Peer review and quality: A dubious connection? *Science*; 293: 2187–88.

Entwistle V A, Renfrew M J, Yearley S, Forrester J, Lamont T (1998). Lay perspectives: Advantages for health research. *BMJ*; 316: 463–66.

EPSRC (2000). *EPSRC concordat with the Department of Health.* London: Engineering and Physical Science Research Council.

Epstein S S (1998). *The politics of cancer revisited.* New York: East Ridge Press.

European Health Management Association (2002). *EU consultation on better medicines for children*; 20; 11 March 2001. www.ehma.org.

Ewald P W (2000). *Plague time.* London: Free Press.

Faulkner W, Senker J, Velho L (1995). *Knowledge frontiers: Public sector research and industrial innovation in biotechnology, engineering ceramics, and parallel computing.* Oxford: Clarendon Press.

Fears R, Poste G, editors (1998). *Radicalism, rationalising or rationing – what does the UK want from research in the science base and health service?* Harlow: SmithKline Beecham Pharmaceuticals.

Ferguson B, Sheldon T, Posnett J, editors (1997). *Concentration and choice in healthcare.* London: Royal Society of Medicine.

Ferlie E, Pettigrew A (1996). Managing through networks: Some issues and implications for the NHS. *British Journal of Management*; 7(special): S81–S99.

Financial Secretary to the Treasury (2000). *Treasury minute on the twentieth to the twenty-fourth reports from the Committee of Public Accounts 1999–2000.* London: HM Treasury.

Financial Times (2001). Europe losing faith in science. *Financial Times* 21 December; 13.

Flagle C D (1992). The integrated health-care system: Reflection and projection. *Journal of the Society for Health Systems*; 3: 16–24.

Forsdyke D R (2000). *Tomorrow's cures today? How to reform the health research system.* Amsterdam: Harwood Academic Publishers.

Foundation for Integrated Medicine (1997). *Integrated healthcare: A way forward for the next five years? A discussion document.* London: Foundation for Integrated Medicine.

Fourcroy J L (1994). *Women and the development of drugs: Why can't a woman be more like a man?* Annals of the New York Academy of Sciences; 736: 174–95.

Francis S, Glanville R (2001). *Building a 2020 vision: Future health care environments.* London: Nuffield Trust and RIBA.

Fraser S W, Greenhalgh T (2001). Coping with complexity: Educating for capability. *BMJ*; 323: 799–803.

Fujimura J (1996). *Crafting science: A sociohistory of the quest for the genetics of cancer.* Cambridge, Mass.: Harvard University Press.

Fuller S (2000). *The governance of science: Ideology and the future of the open society.* Buckingham: Open University Press.

Gelijns A C, Rosenberg N, Moskowitz A J (1998). Capturing the unexpected benefits of medical research. *New England Journal of Medicine*; 339: 693–98.

Global Forum for Health Research (2002). *The 10/90 report on health research 2001/2002.* Downloadable from www.globalforumhealth.org.

Goddard A, Thomson A (2001). Ministers favour RAE elite. *The Times Higher Education Supplement* 21/28 December; 1.

Godlee F, Jefferson T, editors (1999). *Peer review in health sciences.* London: BMJ Books.

Goldberg P (2002). Charity funds for cancer research [letter]. *The Times* 12 February.

Goode A (1994). *The limits of medicine: How science shapes our hopes for the future.* New York: Times Books.

Goodman N W (1999). Who will challenge evidence-based medicine? *Journal of the Royal College of Physicians of London*; 33: 249–51.

Gotzsche PC, Olsen O (2000). Is screening for breast cancer with mammography justified? *Lancet*; 355: 129–34.

Great Britain Parliament (1997). *The new NHS: modern, dependable.* Cm 3807. London: HMSO.

Greenberg D (1997). Washington – keep your hands off, please, NIH tells Congress. *Lancet*; 349: 1821.

Grimley Evans J (1997). A correct compassion: The medical response to an ageing society. *Journal of the Royal College of Physicians of London*; 31: 674–84.

Gross C P *et al* (1999). The relation between funding by the National Institutes of Health and the burden of disease. *New England Journal of Medicine*; 340: 1881–87.

Guillebaud C, chair (1956). *Report of the Committee of Enquiry into the Cost of the National Health Service*. Cmd 9663. London: HMSO.

Guston D H, Keniston K (1994). Introduction: The social contract for science. In: Guston D H, Keniston K, editors. *The fragile contract: University science and the Federal Government*. Cambridge, Mass.: Massachusetts Institute of Technology: 1–41.

Guston D H, Keniston K, editors (1994). *The fragile contract: University science and the Federal Government*. Cambridge, Mass.: Massachusetts Institute of Technology.

Haffner M E (1998). Orphan drug development – International program and study design issues. *Drug Information Journal*; 32: 93–99.

Halpern S (2002). The accidental manager. *British Journal of Health Care Management*; 8: 46–47.

Hamilton G (2001). Dead man walking. *New Scientist* 4/11 August; 31–33.

Hammersley M, Gomm R (1997). Bias in social research. *Sociological Research Online*; 2(1).

Hansmann H (1980). The role of non-profit enterprise. *Yale Law Journal*; 89: 835–901.

Hanson M J, Callahan D (1999). *The goals of medicine: the forgotten issue in health care reform*. Washington: Georgetown University Press.

Hardie J (2001). *Crafting the mental goods*. OpenDemocracy. Accessed at www.open democracy.co.uk

Harrison A (2001). *Making the right connections: The design and management of health care delivery*. London: King's Fund.

Harrison A, Dixon J (2000). *The NHS: Facing the future*. London: King's Fund.

Harrison A, Mulligan J-A (2000). *NHS priorities and needs funding: King's Fund response to consultation paper*. London: King's Fund.

Harvey Brown R (1998). *Towards a democratic science: Scientific narration and civic communication*. New Haven and London: Yale University Press.

Hayek F A (1945). The use of knowledge in society. *The American Economic Review*; XXXV(Four): 518–30.

Haynes M A, Smedley B D, editors (1999). *The unequal burden of cancer: An assessment of NIH research and programs for ethnic minorities and the medically underserved*. Washington DC: National Academy Press.

HEFCE (2001). *Research in nursing and allied health professions*. Higher Education Funding Council for England.

HEFCE (1999). *Good practice in NHS/academic links.* Higher Education Funding Council for England.

HEFCE/JM Consulting (2002a). *Research relationships between higher education institutions and the charitable sector: A report by JM Consulting to the HEFCE on mapping and good practice.* Higher Education Funding Council for England.

HEFCE/JM Consulting (2002b). *Research relationships between higher education institutions and the charitable sector: A report by JM Consulting to the HEFCE on policy.* Higher Education Funding Council for England.

HEFCE/Joint Medical Advisory Committee (1995). *University NHS interactions: A report by the Joint Medical Advisory Committee.* Bristol: Higher Education Funding Council for England.

Help for Health Trust (1999). *Involvement works: The second report of the Standing Group on Consumers in NHS Research.* Winchester: Help for Health Trust.

Henkel M, Kogan M (1981). *The DHSS funded research units: The process of review.* Uxbridge: Brunel University Department of Government.

Hess D J (1999). *Evaluating alternative cancer therapies.* London: Rutgers University Press.

Hess D J (1997). *Can bacteria cause cancer? Alternative medicine confronts big science.* New York and London: New York University Press.

Higgs J, Titchen A (2001). *Practice knowledge and expertise in the health professions.* Oxford: Butterworth–Heinemann.

Horrobin D F (2001). Something rotten at the core of science? *Trends in Pharmacological Science*; 22: 51.

Horrobin D F (1996). Peer review of grant applications. *Lancet*; 348: 1293–95.

Horrobin D F (1990). The philosophical basis of peer review and the suppression of innovation. *JAMA*; 263: 1438–41.

Horton R (2001). Screening mammography – an overview revisited. *Lancet*; 358: 1284–85.

House of Commons Select Committee on Science and Technology (2002). *Cancer research: A follow-up.* London: The Stationery Office.

House of Commons Select Committee on Science and Technology (2000). *Cancer Research: a fresh approach.* London: The Stationery Office.

House of Lords Select Committee on Science and Technology (2000a). *Complementary and alternative medicine.* London: HMSO.

House of Lords Select Committee on Science and Technology (2000b). *Third report: science and society.* Cm 4875. London: The Stationery Office.

House of Lords Select Committee on Science and Technology (1995). *Medical research and the NHS reforms.* London: HMSO.

House of Lords Select Committee on Science and Technology (1988). *Priorities in medical research: Volume 1 – Report.* London: HMSO.

Illich I (1975). *Medical nemesis: the expropriation of health.* London: Calder & Boyars.

Illich I, Zola I K, McKnight J, Caplan J, Shaiken H (1977). *Disabling professions.* London: Marion Boyars Publishers.

Imparato N, editor (1999). *Capital for our time: The economic, legal, and management challenges of intellectual capital.* Stanford, CA: Hoover Institution Press.

Institute of Medicine (1998). *Scientific opportunities and public needs: Improving priority setting and public input at the National Institutes of Health.* Washington DC: National Academy Press.

Jackson C (2001). 'Teaching' primary care trusts – An important development for pharmacy in the future? *Pharmaceutical Journal*; 267: 57–58.

Jenkins-Clarke S *et al* (1997). *Skill mix in primary care: a study of the interface between the general practitioner and other members of the primary health care team. A final report.* York: University of York.

Jevons F R (1973). *Science observed: Science as a social and intellectual activity.* London: George Allen and Unwin.

Jewell D (2001). MMR and the age of unreason. *British Journal of General Practice* November: 875–76.

Johnston K, Sussex J, editors (2000). *Surgical research and development in the NHS – Promotion, management and evaluation.* London: Office of Health Economics.

Jones S (2000). *Genetics in medicine: Real promises, unreal expectations. One scientist's advice to policymakers in the United Kingdom and the United States.* New York: Milbank Memorial Fund.

Kealey T (1996). *The economic laws of scientific research.* Basingstoke: Macmillan.

Kendall J, Knapp M (1996). *The voluntary sector in the United Kingdom.* Manchester: Manchester University Press.

Kennedy I (1981). *Unmasking of medicine.* Oxford: Oxford University Press.

Kennedy I, chair, Bristol Royal Infirmary Public Inquiry, and Great Britain Parliament (2001). *The report of the public inquiry into children's heart surgery at the Bristol Royal Infirmary 1984–1995: learning from Bristol.* Cm 5207(I). Bristol: Bristol Royal Infirmary.

Kerr D J, Edwards B (2000). The Calman-Hine plan and a framework for improving cancer services. In: Appleby J, Harrison A, editors. *Health care UK Autumn 2000.* London: King's Fund.

King's Fund (2000a). *Response to R&D consultation.* London: King's Fund.

King's Fund (2000b). *Age discrimination in health and social services. Notes of a seminar held at the King's Fund on 27 October 2000.* London: King's Fund.

Klein R (1990). Research, policy, and the National Health Service. *Journal of Health Politics, Policy and Law*; 15: 501–23.

Korn D (2000). Conflicts of interest in biomedical research. *JAMA*; 284: 2234–37.

Kremer M (1988). Patent buyouts: a mechanism for encouraging innovation. *Quarterly Journal of Economics*; Nov: 1137–67.

Kuhn T (1962). *The structure of scientific revolutions*. Chicago: University of Chicago Press.

Larkin M (1999). Parkinson's disease research moves on briskly. *Lancet*; 353: 566.

Lazear E P (1999). Intellectual property: A discussion of problems and solutions. In: Imparato N, editor. *Capital for our time: The economic, legal, and management challenges of intellectual capital*. Stanford, CA: Hoover Institution Press: 107–22.

Le Grand J (1991). The theory of Government failure. *British Journal of Political Science*; 21: 423–42.

Lewis J, Ritchie J (1995). *Advancing research*. London: Social and Community Planning Research.

Lichtenberg F R (1999). *Pharmaceutical innovation, mortality reduction, and economic growth*. Washington DC: National Bureau of Economic Research.

Lichtenberg F R (1998). *The allocation of publicly-funded biomedical research*. Working Paper 6601. Cambridge, Mass: National Bureau of Economic Research.

Lichtenberg F R (1996). Do (more and better) drugs keep people out of hospitals? *Health Economics*; 86: 384–88.

Lichtenberg F R, Siegel D (1991). The impact of R&D investment on productivity – New evidence using linked R&D – LRD data. *Economic Inquiry*; XXIX(April): 203–28.

London Implementation Group (1993). *Reports of an independent review of specialist services: cancer*. London: Department of Health.

Long C (1999). Patients and innovation in biotechnology and genomics. In: Imparato N, editor. *Capital for our time: The economic, legal and management challenges of intellectual capital*. Stanford, CA: Hoover Institution Press.

Lord Privy Seal (1972). *Framework for Government research and development*. London: HMSO.

Love J (2000). *Paying for health care R&D: Carrots and sticks*. Accessed at www.cptech.org website.

Lowrance W (1985). *Modern science and human values*. Oxford: Oxford University Press.

Mann J (1999). *The elusive magic bullet: The search for the perfect drug*. Oxford: Oxford University Press.

Martin B (1999). Suppressing research data: Methods, context, accountability, and responses. *Accountability in Research*; 6: 333–72.

Martin B (1979). *The bias of science*. Canberra: Society for Social Responsibility in Science.

Mather S (2000). Cancer research in need of funds [letter]. *The Times* 27 November; 19.

Matterson C (2001). Science must work hard to win back public confidence. *Research Fortnight* 24 October: 17.

Maynard A, Bloor K (1997). Regulating the pharmaceutical industry. *BMJ*; 315: 200–01.

McGeary M, Burstein M (1999). *Sources of cancer research funding in the United States.* Washington DC: National Cancer Policy Board, Institute of Medicine.

McKinlay J, Marceau L (2000). US public health and the 21st century: Diabetes mellitus. *Lancet*; 356: 757–61.

McLachlan G, editor (1990). *What price quality? The NHS in review.* London: Nuffield Provincial Hospitals Trust.

McLachlan G, editor (1985). *A fresh look at policies for health services research and its relevance to management.* London: Nuffield Provincial Hospitals Trust.

McLachlan G, editor (1981). *Matters of moment: management, inner cities, maternity, collaboration.* London: Nuffield Provincial Hospitals Trust.

McLachlan G, editor (1978). *Five years after: A review of health care research management after Rothschild.* London: Nuffield Provincial Hospitals Trust.

McLachlan G, editor (1971). *Portfolio for health: The role and programme of the DHSS in health services research.* London: Nuffield Provincial Hospitals Trust.

Medawar C (1997). The antidepressant web: Marketing depression and making medicines work. *International Journal of Risk & Safety in Medicine*; 10: 75–126.

Melville A, Johnson C (1982). *Cured to death: The effects of prescription drugs.* London: Secker & Warburg.

Melzer D (1998). Health policy and the scientific literature: what kinds of evidence should we expect to find? *Evidence-Based Health Policy and Management*; March: 2–3.

Meltzer D, Johannesson M (1999). Inconsistencies in the 'society perspective' on costs of the Panel on Cost-Effectiveness in Health and Medicine. *Medical Decision Making*; 19: 371–77.

MHA (2002). *Final report: formula.* London: MHA Consultants.

MHA (2000). *NHS support for science R&D activity and cost modelling interim report.* London: MHA Consultants.

Michaud C M, Murray C J L, Bloom B R (2001). Burden of disease – Implications for future research. *JAMA*; 285: 535–39.

Minghetti P, Giudici E M, Montanari L (2000). A proposal to improve the supply of orphan drugs. *Pharmacological Research*; 42: 34–37.

Ministry of Health (1949). Organisation of a regional cancer service. *RHB* (49)92. London: HMSO.

Mohanna K, Chambers R (2001). *Risk matters in healthcare: Communicating, explaining and managing risk.* Oxford: Radcliffe Medical Press.

Moran G (1998). *Silencing scientists and scholars in other fields: Power paradigm controls, peer review, and scholarly communication.* Greenwich, Conn.: Ablex Publishing Corporation.

Morris N (1977). *The cancer blackout: Exposing the official blacklisting of beneficial cancer research, treatment and prevention.* Los Angeles: Regent House.

Moss R W (1996). *The cancer industry.* London: Random.

MRC (2002). *Ageing.* London: Medical Research Council.

MRC (2001). *MRC clinical trials competition.* London: Medical Research Council.

MRC (2000). *A framework for development and evaluation of RCTs for complex interventions to improve health.* London: Medical Research Council.

MRC (1997). *Primary health care 1997.* London: Medical Research Council.

MRC (1994a). *Priorities for health: the research response.* London: Medical Research Council.

MRC (1994b). *The health of the UK's elderly people: MRC review of research issues and opportunities.* London: Medical Research Council.

MRC (1993). *Research developments relevant to NHS practice and health departments policy.* London: Medical Research Council.

MRC (1992). *Concordat between the health departments and the Medical Research Council.* London: Medical Research Council.

Muir Gray J A (1999). Postmodern medicine. *Lancet*; 354: 1552.

Mulligan J (2000). *Why are cancer deaths falling?* King's Fund: London.

Mundy A (2001). *Dispensing with the truth: The victims, the drug companies, and the dramatic story behind the battle over Fen-Phen.* New York: St Martin's Press.

Murray C J L, Lopez A D, editors (1996). *The global burden of disease.* Boston: Harvard School of Public Health.

National Audit Office (2002). *Delivering the commercialisation of public sector science.* London: The Stationery Office.

National Audit Office/NHS Executive (1999). *The management of medical equipment in NHS acute trusts in England.* London: The Stationery Office.

NEJM editorial (1999). Evaluating the burden of disease and spending the research dollars of the National Institutes of Health. *New England Journal of Medicine*; 340: 1914–15.

Neumann P J, Sandberg E A (1998). Trends in health care R&D and technology innovation. *Health Affairs*; 17: 111–18.

New B (1996). The rationing agenda in the NHS. *BMJ*; 312: 1593–1601.

New Scientist editorial (2002). Come clean: Britain's stance on MMR won't wash, and people know it. *New Scientist*; 6 February: 5.

New Scientist editorial (2001). Reality check: A little public scepticism does science no harm. *New Scientist*; 22/29 December, 3.

NHS Executive (1999). *The annual report of the NHS Health Technology Assessment programme 1999.* London: Department of Health.

NHS Executive (1998). *Research: What's in it for consumers? 1st report of the Standing Advisory Group on Consumer Involvement in the NHS R&D Programme to the Central Research & Development Committee 1996/97.* Leeds: NHS Executive.

NHS Executive (1997). *R&D in primary care.* Leeds: NHS Executive.

North East Thames Regional Health Authority (1985). *Review of Cancer Treatment Services.* London: North East Thames RHA.

Nuffield Trust, Working Group on NHS/University Relations (2000). *University clinical partnership: Harnessing clinical and academic resources.* London: Nuffield Trust.

O'Donnell C A, Drummond N, Ross S (1999). Out of hours primary care: A critical overview of current knowledge. *Health Bulletin*; 57: 276–84.

OECD (2001). *Measuring expenditure on health related R&D.* Paris: OECD.

Parkinson's Disease Society of the UK (1999). *Report and financial statements 1999.* London: Parkinson's Disease Society.

Pattison, Professor Sir John, Department of Health (2001). *Modernisation of NHS R&D funding.* Letter. London: Department of Health.

Payne S (1993). Constraints for nursing in developing a framework for cancer care research. *European Journal of Cancer Care*; 2: 117–20.

Peckham S M, editor (1996). *The scientific basis of health services.* London: BMJ Publishing.

Pickles H (1996). Research and development in the new NHS: Another challenge for the profession. *Journal of the Royal College of Physicians of London*; 30: 509–11.

Pickstone J V (2000). *Ways of knowing: A new history of science, technology and medicine.* Chicago: University of Chicago Press.

Plsek P E, Wilson T (2001). Complexity, leadership, and management in healthcare organisations. *BMJ*; 323: 746–49.

Plsek P E, Greenhalgh T (2001). The challenge of complexity in health care. *BMJ*; 323, 625–28.

Porter R J, Malone T E, Vaughan C C, editors (1992). *Biomedical research: Collaboration and conflict of interest.* Baltimore: Johns Hopkins University Press.

Pritchard C, editor (2001). *Capturing the unexpected benefits of medical research.* London: Office of Health Economics.

Proctor R N (1995). *Cancer wars: How politics shapes what we know and don't know about cancer.* New York: Basic Books.

Rafferty A-M, Traynor M (2000). *Measuring the outputs of nursing R&D.* London: London School of Hygiene and Tropical Medicine.

Rafferty A-M, Traynor M (1998). *Nursing, research and the higher education context: A second working paper.* London: London School of Hygiene and Tropical Medicine.

Resnik D (1999). Conflicts of interest in science. *Perspectives on Science*; 6: 381–408.

Resnik D (1998). Industry-sponsored research: Secrecy versus corporate responsibility. *Business and Society Review*; 99: 31–34.

Roberts E, Robinson J, Seymour L (2002). *Old habits die hard: Tackling age discrimination in health and social care.* London: King's Fund.

Roberts, Sir Gareth, chair (2002). *SET for success: The supply of people with science, technology, engineering and mathematics skills.* London: The Stationery Office.

Rosser Matthews J (1995). *Quantification and the quest for medical certainty.* Princeton, NJ: Princeton University Press.

Rothschild, Lord (1971). The organization and management of Government research and development. As Head of the Central Policy Review Staff. In *A framework for Government research and development.* Cmnd 4814. London: HMSO.

Rothwell P M (2001). The high cost of not funding stroke research: a comparison with heart disease and cancer. *Lancet*; 357: 1612–16.

Royal Pharmaceutical Society of Great Britain (2001). *IPPR Commission on Public Private Partnerships: Call for evidence. RPSGB Submission in Respect to Section III Q 21–23.* London: Royal Pharmaceutical Society of Great Britain.

Royal Pharmaceutical Society of Great Britain (1999). *Medicines, pharmacy and the NHS: Getting it right for patients and prescribers. Setting the clinical effectiveness agenda for pharmacy.* London: Royal Pharmaceutical Society of Great Britain.

Royal Pharmaceutical Society of Great Britain (1997). *A new age for pharmacy practice research: Promoting evidence-based practice in pharmacy.* London: Royal Pharmaceutical Society of Great Britain.

Saks M (1995). *Professions and the public interest: Medical power, altruism and alternative medicine.* London: Routledge.

Savill, Sir John, chair (2000). *The tenure-track clinician scientist: A new career pathway to promote recruitment into clinical academic medicine.* London: Academy of Medical Sciences.

Schwart M, Thompson M (1990). *Divided we stand: Redefining politics, technology and social choice.* Philadelphia: University of Pennsylvania Press.

Shulman S R, Manocchia M (1997). The US Orphan Drug Programme 1983–1995. *Pharmacoeconomics*; 12: 312–26.

SmithKline Beecham (1999). *Health matters! How will science deliver on its promise to improve healthcare?*

Smith P, editor (1998). *Nursing research: Setting new agendas.* London: Arnold.

Smith R (1999). The future of peer review. In Godlee F, Jefferson T, editors. *Peer review in health sciences*, London: BMJ Books.

Smith T (2001). *University clinical partnership: A new framework for NHS/university relations.* London: The Stationery Office and Nuffield Trust.

Spece R G Jr, Shimm D S, Buchanan A E (1996). *Conflicts of interest in clinical practice and research.* Oxford: Oxford University Press.

Standing Advisory Group on Consumer Involvement in the NHS Research and Development Programme (1998). *Research: What's in it for me? Conference report.* London: Department of Health.

Steering Group on Undergraduate Medical and Dental Education and Research (1996). *Undergraduate Medical and Dental Education and Research: Fourth Report of the Steering Group.* London: Department of Health.

Stevens R (1998). *American medicine and the public interest.* London: University of California Press.

Stewart G (1999). *The partnership between science and industry: Co-operation or conflict of interest?* London: The British Library.

Stowe K (1989). *On caring for the national health.* London; Nuffield Provincial Hospitals Trust.

Sulston J, Ferry G (2002). *The common thread: A story of science, politics, ethics and the human genome.* London: Bantam Press.

Scottish Universities Research Policy Consortium (2002). *University research in Scotland: Developing a policy framework.* Edinburgh, Scottish Universities Research Policy Consortium.

Swales J D (1997). Science in a health service. *Lancet*; 349: 1319–21.

Swales J D (1996). NHS letter to the chief executive of trusts. 31 July.

Swales J D (1995). *The growth of medical science: The lessons of Malthus.* London: Royal College of Physicians of London.

Sweeney K G *et al* (1998). Personal significance: the third dimension. *Lancet*; 351: 134–36.

Sykes R B (2000). *New medicines: The practice of medicine and public policy.* London: Nuffield Trust.

Tallon D, Chard J, Dieppe P (2000). Relation between agendas of the research community and the research consumer. *Lancet*; 355: 2037–40.

Tanenbaum S J (1993). What physicians know. *New England Journal of Medicine*; 21 October: 1268–70.

Tavakoli M, Davies H T O, Malek M, editors (2001). *Health policy and economics: Strategic issues in health care management.* Aldershot: Ashgate.

Ten Have H A, Kimsma G K, Spicker S F (1990). *The growth of medical knowledge.* Dordrecht, The Netherlands: Kluwer Academic Publishers.

Thamer M, Brennan N, Semansky R (1998). A cross-national comparison of orphan drug policies: Implications for the U.S. Orphan Drug Act. *Journal of Health Politics, Policy and Law*; 23: 265–90.

Thomson H, Petticrew M, Morrison D (2001). Health effect of housing improvement: systematic review of intervention studies. *BMJ*; 323: 187–90.

Thurow Lester C, editor (1999). *Creating wealth: The new rules for individuals, companies, and countries in a knowledge-based economy.* London: Nicholas Brealey Publishing.

Tomlinson, Sir Bernard, chair (1992). *Report of the Inquiry into London's Health Service, Medical Education and Research.* London: HMSO.

Trinder L (2000). A critical appraisal of evidence-based practice. In: Trinder L, Reynolds S, editors. *Evidence-based practice: A critical appraisal.* Oxford: Blackwell Sciences, 212–41.

Trinder L, Reynolds S, editors (2000). *Evidence-based practice: A critical appraisal.* Oxford: Blackwell Sciences.

Tversky A, Kahneman D (1982). Judgement under uncertainty: heuristics and biases. In: Kahneman D, Slovic P, Tversky A, editors. *Judgement under uncertainty.* Cambridge: Cambridge University Press.

Wanless, Sir Derek (2001). *Securing our future health: Taking a long term view.* London: The Stationery Office.

Weatherall D (1995). *Science and the quiet art: The role of medical research in health care.* Oxford: W W Norton & Co.

Weinstein M C *et al* (1987). Forecasting coronary heart disease incidence, mortality, and cost: The coronary heart disease policy model. *American Journal of Public Health*; 77: 1417–25.

Weisbrod B (1977). *The voluntary non-profit sector: An economic analysis.* Mass.: Lexington Books.

Wellcome News (2000). Questioning the alternative: Scientific assessment of complementary and alternative therapies. *Wellcome News*; 23: 10–11.

Wenger N K (1992). Exclusion of the elderly and women from coronary trials: Is their quality of care compromised? *JAMA*; 268: 1460–61.

West R (1991). *Parkinson's disease.* London: Office of Health Economics.

Wheeler P (2000). Private investigation. *Hospital Doctor*; February: 21–23.

Whelan J (1998), Age Concern England. *Equal access to cardiac rehabilitation: Age discrimination in the NHS – cardiac rehabilitation services.* London: Age Concern England.

White House (2002), *Commission on Complementary and Alternative Medicine Policy. Final Report.* March. www.whccamp.hhs.gov

Wilson T, Holt T (2001). Complexity and social care. *BMJ*; 323: 685–88.

Wood B (2000). Patient power? *The politics of patients' associations in Britain and America.* Buckingham: Open University Press.

Working Group on Priority Setting (1997). *Setting research priorities at the National Institutes of Health.* Bethesda, Md: National Institutes of Health.

Wright P, Treacher A, editors (1982). *The problem of medical knowledge: Examining the social construction of medicine.* Edinburgh: Edinburgh University Press.

Index

Page numbers in *italics* refer to tables; *n* indicates notes; *passim* indicates numerous intermittent references within page ranges.